Ovarian Cancer

LEARNING that you have cancer can be overwhelming.

The goal of this book is to help you get the best care. It explains which tests and treatments are recommended by experts in ovarian cancer.

The National Comprehensive Cancer Network® (NCCN®) is a not-for-profit alliance of 27 leading cancer centers. Experts from NCCN have written treatment guidelines for doctors who treat ovarian cancer. These treatment guidelines suggest what the best practice is for cancer care. The information in this patient book is based on the guidelines written for doctors.

This book focuses on the treatment of ovarian cancer. Key points of the book are summarized in the NCCN Quick Guide™ series for ovarian cancer. NCCN also offers patient books on breast cancer, lung cancer, melanoma, and many other cancer types. Visit NCCN.org/patients for the full library of patient books, summaries, and other resources.

WM. BEAUMONT HOSPITAL
CANCER RESOURCE CENTER
3577 W. 13 MILE RD.
ROYAL OAK, MI 48073
(248) 551-1339

"This material is intended to provide general information to you. Consult your health care professional with any questions relating to a medical problem or condition."

About

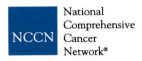

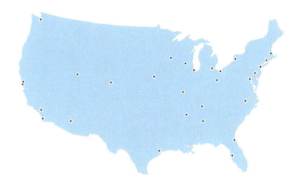

These patient guidelines for cancer care are produced by the National Comprehensive Cancer Network® (NCCN®).

The mission of NCCN is to improve cancer care so people can live better lives. At the core of NCCN are the NCCN Clinical Practice Guidelines in Oncology (NCCN Guidelines®). NCCN Guidelines® contain information to help health care workers plan the best cancer care. They list options for cancer care that are most likely to have the best results. The NCCN Guidelines for Patients® present the information from the NCCN Guidelines in an easy-to-learn format.

Panels of experts create the NCCN Guidelines. Most of the experts are from NCCN Member Institutions. Their areas of expertise are diverse. Many panels also include a patient advocate. Recommendations in the NCCN Guidelines are based on clinical trials and the experience of the panelists. The NCCN Guidelines are updated at least once a year. When funded, the patient books are updated to reflect the most recent version of the NCCN Guidelines for doctors.

For more information about the NCCN Guidelines, visit NCCN.org/clinical.asp.

Dorothy A. Shead, MS
Director, Patient and Clinical Information Operations

Laura J. Hanisch, PsyD
Medical Writer/Patient Information Specialist

Rachael Clarke
Guidelines Data and Layout Coordinator

Alycia Corrigan
Medical Writer

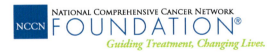

NCCN Foundation was founded by NCCN to raise funds for patient education based on the NCCN Guidelines. NCCN Foundation offers guidance to people with cancer and their caregivers at every step of their cancer journey. This is done by sharing key information from leading cancer experts. This information can be found in a library of NCCN Guidelines for Patients® and other patient education resources. NCCN Foundation is also committed to advancing cancer treatment by funding the nation's promising doctors at the center of cancer research, education, and progress of cancer therapies.

For more information about NCCN Foundation, visit NCCNFoundation.org.

© 2017 National Comprehensive Cancer Network, Inc. Posted 06/28/2017.

All rights reserved. NCCN Guidelines for Patients® and illustrations herein may not be reproduced in any form for any purpose without the express written permission of NCCN. The NCCN Guidelines are a work in progress that may be redefined as often as new significant data becomes available. The NCCN makes no warranties of any kind whatsoever regarding their content, use, or application and disclaims any responsibility for their application or use in any way.

National Comprehensive Cancer Network (NCCN) • 275 Commerce Drive, Suite 300 • Fort Washington, PA 19034 • 215.690.0300

Supporters

Endorsed and sponsored in part by

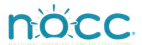

National Ovarian Cancer Coalition
The National Ovarian Cancer Coalition® is pleased to have provided critical funding necessary to ensure the production of the NCCN Patient Guidelines. We believe the guidelines are an important resource that informs patients and promotes best practices for healthcare professionals, and aligns with our mission "to save lives by fighting tirelessly to prevent and cure ovarian cancer and to improve the quality of life for survivors." For support or more information about our history and groundbreaking work to empower the community, please visit www.ovarian.org or call us at 1-888-OVARIAN. www.ovarian.org

Endorsed by

Ovarian Cancer Research Fund Alliance (OCRFA)
As the largest ovarian cancer research, advocacy and patient support organization, Ovarian Cancer Research Fund Alliance commends NCCN for providing such an important and useful resource to our community. ocrfa.org

The Society of Gynecologic Oncology (SGO)
The Society of Gynecologic Oncology (SGO) fully endorses the NCCN Guidelines for Patients: Ovarian Cancer. SGO urges individuals who suspect they have a gynecologic cancer, or who have been so diagnosed, to seek treatment from a gynecologic oncologist, a physician who specializes in diagnosing and treating cancers that are located on the reproductive organs. sgo.org

Foundation for Women's Cancer
The Foundation for Women's Cancer is pleased to support this comprehensive resource for patients and their families. It is especially important for women to be aware of their risks and symptoms for this cancer, as well as treatment options, including care by a gynecologic oncologist. foundationforwomenscancer.org

Sharsheret
Sharsheret is proud to endorse this important resource, the NCCN Guidelines for Patients: Ovarian Cancer. With this critical tool in hand, women nationwide have the knowledge they need to partner with their healthcare team to navigate the often complicated world of ovarian cancer care and make informed treatment decisions. sharsheret.org

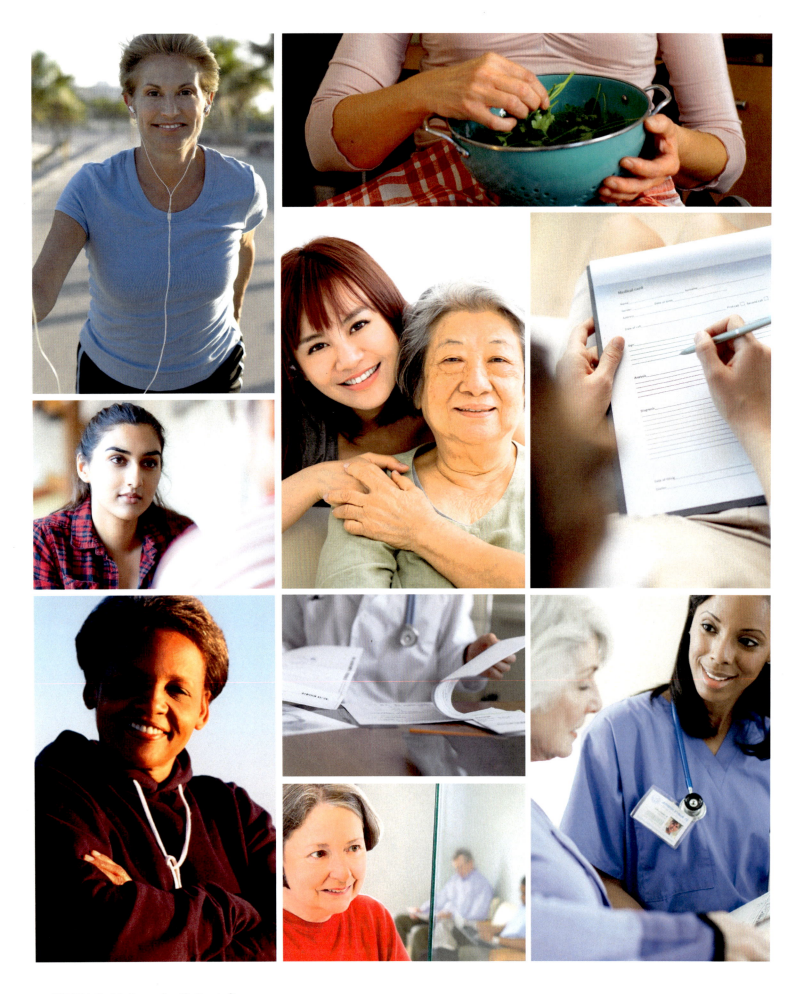

Ovarian Cancer

Contents

6   How to use this book

7   Part 1
    Ovarian cancer
    Explains where ovarian cancer starts, how it spreads, and the symptoms it may cause.

13 Part 2
    Testing for ovarian cancer
    Describes the tests doctors use to find and confirm (diagnose) ovarian cancer and plan treatment.

22 Part 3
    Cancer staging
    Explains how doctors assess and rate the extent of ovarian cancer in your body.

34 Part 4
    Overview of cancer treatments
    Describes the treatments that are used for ovarian cancer.

44 Part 5
    Treatment guide for epithelial ovarian cancer
    Presents the recommended course of action for epithelial ovarian cancer from diagnosis to after cancer treatment.

63 Part 6
    Treatment guide for LCOH (less common types of ovarian histopathologies)
    Presents the recommended course of action for less common types of ovarian cancer from diagnosis to after cancer treatment.

81 Part 7
    Making treatment decisions
    Offers tips for getting a treatment plan that meets all your needs.

88 Glossary
    Dictionary
    Acronyms

98 NCCN Panel Members

99 NCCN Member Institutions

100 Index

How to use this book

Who should read this book?

This book is about treatment for epithelial ovarian cancer—the most common type of ovarian cancer. It also discusses treatment for other less common types of ovarian cancer like borderline epithelial ovarian cancer. Options are also briefly presented in this book for benign (not cancer) tumors of the ovary.

Patients and those who support them—caregivers, family, and friends—may find this book helpful. It may help you talk with your treatment team, understand what doctors say, and prepare for treatment.

Are the book chapters in a certain order?

Early chapters introduce you to the diagnosis and testing for ovarian cancer. Thus, it is helpful to start with **Part 1** of the book. This first chapter discusses how this cancer grows and how it may affect the female body. Tests that help doctors plan treatment are described in **Part 2**. It is important to know the stage of the cancer. Your treatment plan will be partly based on the cancer stage. You can learn more about cancer staging in **Part 3**.

An overview of treatments for ovarian cancer is presented in **Part 4**. Knowing what a treatment is will help you understand your options. Treatment options are presented in **Parts 5 and 6**. Tips for talking with your doctor and helpful online resources are addressed in **Part 7**.

Does this book include all options?

This book includes information for many people. Your treatment team can point out what applies to you. They can also give you more information. While reading, make a list of questions to ask your doctors.

The treatment options are based on science and the experience of NCCN experts. However, their recommendations may not be right for you. Your doctors may suggest other options based on your health and other factors. If other options are given, ask your treatment team questions.

Help! What do the words mean?

In this book, many medical words are included. These are words that your treatment team may say to you. Most of these words may be new to you. It may be a lot to learn.

Don't be discouraged as you read. Keep reading and review the information. Ask your treatment team to explain a word or phrase that you do not understand.

Words that you may not know are defined in the text or in the *Dictionary*. Acronyms are also defined when first used and in the *Glossary*. Acronyms are short words formed from the first letters of several words. One example is DNA for **d**eoxyribo**n**ucleic **a**cid.

1 Ovarian cancer

8 The ovaries
9 Ovarian cancer
10 Cancer cells
12 Symptoms
12 Review

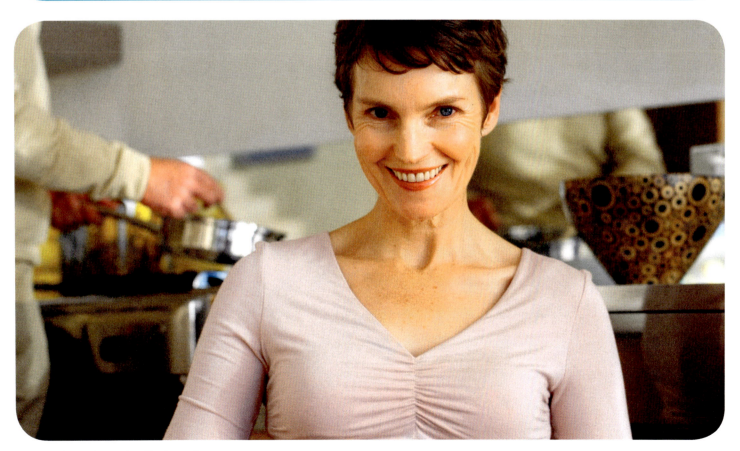

1 Ovarian cancer | The ovaries

Learning that you have cancer can be overwhelming and confusing. Part 1 explains some basics about ovarian cancer that may help you better understand this disease. This information may also help you start planning for treatment.

The ovaries

The ovaries are a pair of organs that are part of the reproductive system in women (females). The reproductive system is the group of organs that work together to make babies. In women, this system includes the ovaries, fallopian tubes, uterus, cervix, and vagina. Each ovary is about the size and shape of a grape. They are located in the pelvis—the area below the belly (abdomen) between the hip bones. One ovary is on the left side of the uterus and one is on the right. Each ovary is connected to the uterus by a long, thin tube called a fallopian tube. **See Figure 1.**

Figure 1
The female reproductive system

The reproductive system is a group of organs that work together to make babies. The female reproductive system includes the ovaries, fallopian tubes, uterus, cervix, and vagina.

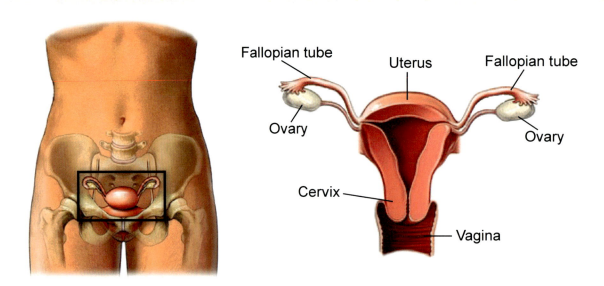

Illustration Copyright © 2017 Nucleus Medical Media, All rights reserved. www.nucleusinc.com

1 Ovarian cancer

The ovaries make eggs for reproduction (making babies). They also make female hormones that affect breast growth, body shape, and the menstrual cycle. Eggs pass out of the ovary and travel through the attached fallopian tube into the uterus. The uterus is where babies grow during pregnancy. It is also called the womb. At least one ovary and the uterus are needed for a woman to have a menstrual cycle and be able to become pregnant.

Ovarian cancer

Cancer is a disease of cells—the building blocks that form tissue in the body. Inside all cells are coded instructions for making new cells and controlling how cells behave. These coded instructions are called genes. Abnormal changes in genes can turn normal ovarian cells into cancer cells.

Normal cells grow and divide to make new cells. New cells are made as the body needs them to replace injured or dying cells. When normal cells grow old or get damaged, they die. Cancer cells don't do this. The changes in genes cause cancer cells to make too many copies of themselves. **See Figure 2.**

Figure 2
Normal versus cancer cell growth

Normal cells divide to make new cells as the body needs them. Normal cells die once they get old or damaged. Cancer cells make new cells that aren't needed and don't die quickly when old or damaged.

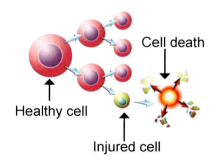
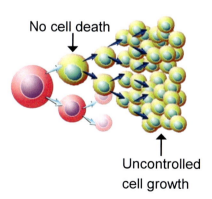

Illustration Copyright © 2017 Nucleus Medical Media, All rights reserved. www.nucleusinc.com

1 Ovarian cancer | Cancer cells

Cancer cells make new cells that aren't needed and don't die quickly when old or damaged. Over time, cancer cells grow and divide enough to form a mass called a tumor. The first tumor formed by the overgrowth of cancer cells is called the primary tumor.

Types of ovarian cancer

The ovaries are made up of three main types of cells: epithelial cells, stromal cells, and germ cells. Cancer can start in each type of cell. Thus, there is more than one type of ovarian cancer.

Most ovarian cancers start in the epithelial cells. This is called epithelial ovarian cancer. Epithelial cells form the outer layer of tissue around the ovary. This layer of tissue is called the epithelium. **See Figure 3.** About 90 out of 100 ovarian cancers are epithelial ovarian cancer. Because it is the most common type, it is often simply referred to as ovarian cancer.

Borderline epithelial tumors [LMP (**l**ow **m**alignant **p**otential] also start in the epithelial cells. It is a rare type of epithelial ovarian cancer. LMP tumors don't grow into the supporting tissue of the ovary. The tumor cells may spread and grow on the surface of nearby organs and tissues. But, they almost never grow into (invade) tissue the way fully cancerous cells do.

This guideline also discusses other LCOH (**l**ess **c**ommon **o**varian **h**istopathologies) including carcinosarcomas (MMMTs [**m**alignant **m**ixed **M**üllerian **t**umors) of the ovary, clear cell carcinomas, mucinous carcinomas, low-grade (grade 1) serous carcinomas/endometrioid epithelial carcinomas, malignant sex cord-stromal tumors, and malignant germ cell tumors.

It is helpful to understand that the terms carcinoma and malignant both refer to cancer when used in the names of the LCOH. The term carcinoma means cancer that starts in the cells that form glands or the lining or organs. Malignant is also used in the names and also means cancer.

Cancer cells

Cancer cells act differently than normal cells in three key ways. First, cancer cells grow without control. Unlike normal cells, cancer cells make new cells that aren't needed and don't die when they should. The cancer cells build up to form a primary tumor.

Second, cancer cells can grow into (invade) other tissues. This is called invasion. Normal cells don't do this. Over time, the primary tumor can grow large and invade tissues outside the ovary. Ovarian cancer often invades the fallopian tubes and uterus.

Third, cancer cells don't stay in one place as they should. Unlike normal cells, cancer cells can spread to other parts of the body. This process is called metastasis. Ovarian cancer cells can break off (shed) from the primary tumor to form new tumors on the surface of nearby organs and tissues. These are called "implants" or "seeds." Implants that grow into supporting tissues of nearby organs are called invasive implants.

Cancer cells can also spread through blood or lymph vessels. Lymph is a clear fluid that gives cells water and food. It also has white blood cells that help fight germs. It travels in small tubes (vessels) to lymph nodes. Lymph nodes are small groups of disease-fighting cells that remove germs from lymph. Lymph vessels and nodes are found all over the body. **See Figure 4.**

1 Ovarian cancer | Cancer cells

Figure 3
Epithelial ovarian cancer

Most ovarian cancers start in the epithelial cells. Epithelial cells form the outer layer of tissue around the ovary. This layer of tissue is called the epithelium. Cancer that starts in these cells is called epithelial ovarian cancer.

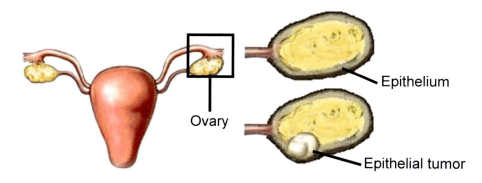

Illustration Copyright © 2017 Nucleus Medical Media, All rights reserved. www.nucleusinc.com

Figure 4
Lymph vessels and nodes

Lymph vessels and nodes are found all over the body. Lymph nodes are small groups of special disease-fighting cells. Lymph nodes are connected to each other by a network of small tubes called lymph vessels.

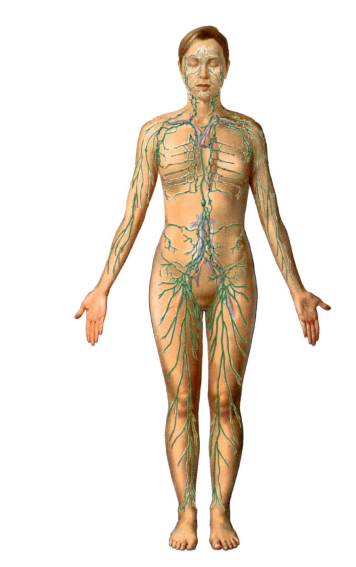

Illustration Copyright © 2017 Nucleus Medical Media, All rights reserved. www.nucleusinc.com

1 Ovarian cancer | Symptoms | Review

The uncontrolled growth, invasion, and spread of cancer cells makes cancer dangerous. But, LMP tumors are less dangerous than other forms of epithelial ovarian cancer. This is because LMP tumors grow on the surface of organs and rarely grow into (invade) normal tissue.

Symptoms

One way to find ovarian cancer early is to know the symptoms of the cancer. Symptoms are health problems that you report to your doctor. Doctors have outlined a set of symptoms that are often seen in women with ovarian cancer. Ovarian cancer may cause certain symptoms early or as it grows larger. The most common symptoms of ovarian cancer include:

- Feeling bloated
- Pain in the pelvis or belly (abdomen)
- Trouble eating or feeling full fast
- Feeling the need to urinate often or urgently

These symptoms can also be caused by many other common health conditions. But, ovarian cancer is more likely to be the cause of these symptoms if they are:

- New and began less than 1 year ago
- Frequent and occur more than 12 days each month

If this describes you, tell your doctor about your symptoms. However, ovarian cancer does not always cause symptoms. Or, ovarian cancer may not cause symptoms until it has grown very large or has spread.

Your doctor may also think you have ovarian cancer based on certain signs. Signs of ovarian cancer include feeling a mass in your pelvis or fluid buildup in your abdomen. Your doctor may feel a mass in your pelvis because of a tumor or enlarged ovary. Ovarian cancer can also cause excess fluid buildup (ascites) in your pelvis and abdomen. This can cause swelling and make your abdomen look or feel enlarged.

Your doctor may suspect ovarian cancer based on these signs and symptoms. But, many other health conditions could be the cause. Therefore, your doctor will give more tests and exams to confirm or rule out ovarian cancer. This is described next in Part 2.

Review

- The ovaries are a pair of organs that make eggs for reproduction (making babies). They also make hormones.
- Ovarian cancer often starts in the cells that form the outer layer of tissue around the ovaries. This is called epithelial ovarian cancer.
- Borderline epithelial tumors (LMP [low malignant potential] also start in the epithelial cells.
- Cancer cells form a tumor since they don't die as they should.
- Cancer cells can break away from the first (primary) tumor and spread to other tissues and organs in the body (metastasis).
- Ovarian cancer may cause symptoms such as: feeling bloated, pain in the belly or pelvis, trouble eating, and needing to urinate often or urgently.

2 Testing for ovarian cancer

15 General health tests
16 Imaging tests
20 Blood tests
21 Tissue tests
21 Review

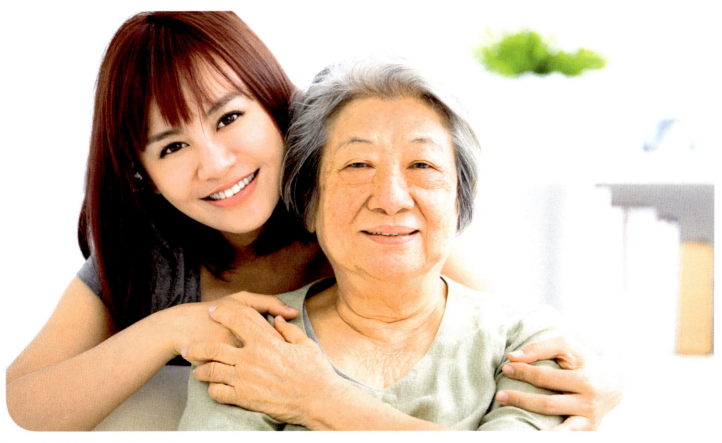

2 Testing for ovarian cancer | General health tests

Part 2 describes the tests that are recommended for ovarian cancer. These tests are used to find and confirm (diagnose) ovarian cancer and plan treatment. They are also used to monitor your health and check treatment results.

Your doctor may suspect ovarian cancer if you have certain symptoms. Or, ovarian cancer may have been found by a prior surgery. To confirm (diagnose) ovarian cancer and plan treatment, a number of tests are needed. Guide 1 lists the different types of tests that are used for ovarian cancer. Read the next pages to learn more about these tests, including when and why each test is recommended. Some tests are done at the initial visit, while other tests are done soon after a diagnosis. It is helpful to ask your doctor which tests you will have and when you can expect the results.

Guide 1. Tests

Type of test	Recommended tests
General health tests	• Family and medical history • Genetic counseling and testing • Check nutritional status • Abdominal and pelvic exam
Blood tests	• CBC (**c**omplete **b**lood **c**ount) • Blood chemistry profile with liver function tests • Total serum protein • CA-125 (**c**ancer **a**ntigen **125**) and other tumor markers
Imaging tests	• Ultrasound • CT (**c**omputed **t**omography) scan of the abdomen and pelvis • MRI (**m**agnetic **r**esonance **i**maging) scan of the abdomen and pelvis • Chest x-ray or CT scan of the chest • GI (**g**astro**i**ntestinal) evaluation
Tissue tests	• Biopsy • Review of tumor tissue

2 Testing for ovarian cancer | General health tests

General health tests

Medical and family history
Your medical history includes any health events in your life and any medications you've taken. Your doctors will want to know about all your illnesses, symptoms, and any prior tests or surgeries. It may help to make a list of old and new medications while at home to bring to your doctor's office.

Ovarian cancer and other health conditions can run in families. Therefore, your doctors will also ask about the medical history of your blood relatives. It's important to know who in your family has had what diseases. It's also important to know at what ages the diseases started. This information is called a family history.

While taking your medical and family history, your doctor may also ask you questions about your nutrition. He or she will want to know about your diet. It is important to follow a healthy diet. This is true for any cancer diagnosis. Tell your doctor or nurse about your eating habits. If you need help with keeping a healthy diet or have questions about your diet, ask your doctor for a referral to a registered dietitian.

Genetic counseling and testing
Ovarian cancer often occurs for unknown reasons. But, about 15 out of 100 ovarian cancers are due to changes in genes that are passed down from a parent to a child. This is called hereditary ovarian cancer. Using your age, medical history, and family history, your doctor will assess how likely you are to have hereditary ovarian cancer.

NCCN experts also recommend genetic counseling for all women diagnosed with ovarian cancer. Genetic counseling is a discussion with a health expert about the risk for a disease caused by changes in genes. This should be led by someone with a lot of experience and expertise such as a genetic counselor.

A genetic counselor has special training to help patients understand changes in genes that are related to disease. The genetic counselor can tell you more about how likely you are to have hereditary ovarian cancer. He or she may suggest genetic testing to look for changes in genes that increase the chances of developing ovarian cancer.

Hereditary ovarian cancer is most often caused by changes (mutations) in the *BRCA1* and *BRCA2* genes. Families with a history of Lynch syndrome (HNPCC [**h**ereditary **n**on**p**olyposis **c**olorectal **c**ancer syndrome]) may also be at risk ovarian cancer as well as other cancers. Both *BRCA* gene mutations and Lynch syndrome put woman at risk for ovarian cancer starting at an early age. When normal, these genes help prevent abnormal cell growth by repairing damaged cells. Genetic testing can tell if you have a mutation in the *BRCA* genes or other genes important in hereditary cancer. See pages 40 and 60 for more on genetic mutations and treatment.

Abdominal and pelvic exam
Doctors often give a physical exam along with taking a medical history. A physical exam is a review of your body for signs of disease. During this exam, your doctor will listen to your lungs, heart, and intestines to assess your general health. He or she will also look at and touch parts of your body to check for abnormal changes.

Your doctor will also give a physical exam of your belly (abdomen) and pelvis—the area between your hip bones. This is called an abdominal and pelvic exam.

For the abdominal exam, your doctor will feel different parts of your belly. This is to see if organs are of normal size, are soft or hard, or cause pain when touched.

Your doctor will also feel for signs of fluid buildup, called ascites. Ascites may be found in the belly area or around the ovaries.

2 Testing for ovarian cancer | Imaging tests

During the pelvic exam, your doctor will feel for abnormal changes in the size, shape, or position of your ovaries and uterus. A special widening instrument will be used to view your vagina and cervix. A sample may be taken for a Pap test at this time.

Imaging tests

Imaging tests take pictures (images) of the inside of your body. Doctors use imaging tests to check if there is a tumor in your ovaries. The pictures can show the tumor size, shape, and location. They can also show if the cancer has spread beyond your ovaries. Different types of imaging tests are used to look for ovarian cancer, plan treatment, and check treatment results.

Getting an imaging test is often easy. Before the test, you may be asked to stop eating or drinking for a few hours. You may also need to remove metal objects from your body. The types of imaging tests used for ovarian cancer are described next.

Ultrasound

An ultrasound is a test that uses sound waves to take pictures of the inside of the body. It is often the first imaging test given to look for ovarian cancer. Ultrasound is good at showing the size, shape, and location of the ovaries, fallopian tubes, uterus, and nearby tissues. It can also show if there is a mass in the ovary and whether the mass is solid or filled with fluid.

This test uses a hand-held device called an ultrasound probe. The probe sends out sound waves that bounce off organs and tissues to make echoes. The probe also picks up the echoes. A computer uses the echoes to make a picture that is shown on a screen. There are two types of ultrasounds that may be used to look for ovarian cancer: transabdominal ultrasound and transvaginal ultrasound.
See Figure 5.

2 Testing for ovarian cancer | Imaging tests

For a transabdominal ultrasound, a gel will be spread on the area of skin near your ovaries. This includes your belly (abdomen) and the area between your hip bones (pelvis). The gel helps to make the pictures clearer. Your doctor will place the probe on your skin and guide it back and forth in the gel.

For a transvaginal ultrasound, your doctor will insert the probe into your vagina. This may help the doctor see your ovaries more clearly. Ultrasounds are generally painless.

But, you may feel a little discomfort when the probe is inserted for a transvaginal ultrasound. An ultrasound can take between 20 and 60 minutes to complete. More or less time may be needed depending on the area of your body being looked at.

An ultrasound uses sound waves to make pictures of the inside of the body. An ultrasound probe sends out the sound waves. For a transabdominal ultrasound, the probe will be placed on the skin of your belly. For a transvaginal ultrasound, it will be inserted into your vagina.

Figure 5
Ultrasound

An ultrasound uses sound waves to make pictures of the inside of the body. An ultrasound probe sends out the sound waves. For a transabdominal ultrasound, the probe will be placed on the skin of your belly. For a transvaginal ultrasound, it will be inserted into your vagina.

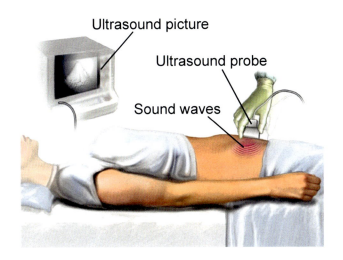
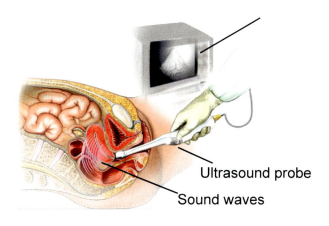

Illustration Copyright © 2017 Nucleus Medical Media, All rights reserved. www.nucleusinc.com

CT scan

A CT scan uses x-rays to take pictures of the inside of the body. It takes many x-rays of the same body part from different angles. All the x-ray pictures are combined to make one detailed picture of the body part.

A CT scan of your chest, abdomen, and/or pelvis may be given along with other initial tests to look for ovarian cancer. This type of scan is good at showing if the cancer has spread outside of the ovaries. But, it is not good at showing small tumors. A CT scan may also show if nearby lymph nodes are bigger than normal, which can be a sign of cancer spread.

Before the CT scan, you may be given a contrast dye to make the pictures clearer. The dye may be put in a glass of water for you to drink, injected into your vein, or both. It may cause you to feel flushed or get hives. Rarely, serious allergic reactions occur. Tell your doctors if you have had bad reactions in the past.

A CT scan machine is large and has a tunnel in the middle. **See Figure 6.** During the scan, you will need to lie face up on a table that moves through the tunnel. The scanner will rotate an x-ray beam around you to take pictures from many angles. You may hear buzzing, clicking, or whirring sounds during this time.

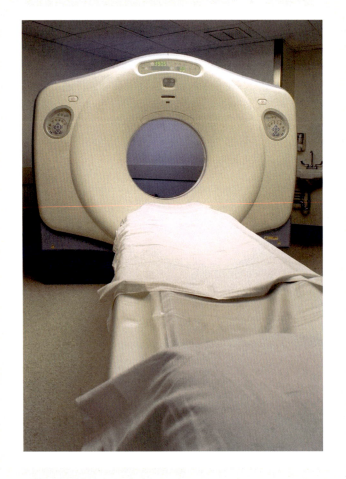

**Figure 6
CT scan machine**

A CT machine is large and has a tunnel in the middle. During the test, you will lie on a table that moves slowly through the tunnel.

2 Testing for ovarian cancer | Imaging tests

One x-ray scan is completed in about 30 seconds. But, the full exam may take 15 to 60 minutes to complete. More or less time may be needed depending on the part of your body being scanned. A computer will combine all the x-ray pictures into one detailed picture. You may not learn of the results for a few days since a radiologist needs to see the pictures. A radiologist is a doctor who's an expert in reading the pictures from imaging tests.

MRI scan
An MRI scan uses radio waves and powerful magnets to take pictures of the inside of the body. It does not use x-rays. This type of scan is good at showing the spine and soft tissues like the brain.

An MRI scan of your abdomen and pelvis may be used to look for ovarian cancer if the ultrasound was unclear. An MRI scan of your chest may be used to look for signs of cancer spread. This test may also be used to check treatment results and to assess for cancer spread to other parts of the body.

Getting an MRI scan is similar to getting a CT scan. But, MRI scans take longer to complete. The full exam can take an hour or more. For the scan, you will need to lie on a table that moves through a large tunnel in the scanning machine. The scan may cause your body to feel a bit warm. Like a CT scan, a contrast dye may be used to make the pictures clearer. You may not learn of the results for a few days since a radiologist needs to see and interpret the pictures.

PET scan
A PET (positron emission tomography) scan shows how your cells are using a simple form of sugar. To create pictures, a sugar radiotracer first needs to be put into your body with an injection into a vein.

The radiotracer emits a small amount of energy that is detected by the machine that takes pictures. Active cancer cells use sugar faster than normal cells. Thus, cancer cells look brighter in the pictures.

PET is very good at showing small groups of cancer cells. This test may also be useful for showing if ovarian cancer has spread. Sometimes, PET is combined with CT—called a PET/CT scan.

Chest x-ray
An x-ray uses small amounts of radiation to make pictures of organs and tissues inside the body. A tumor changes the way radiation is absorbed and will show up on the x-ray picture. A chest x-ray can be used to show if cancer has spread to your lungs. This test may be given with other initial tests when ovarian cancer is first suspected or found. It may also be given after treatment to check treatment results. A chest x-ray is painless and takes about 20 minutes to complete.

GI evaluation
The GI tract is made of the organs that food passes through when you eat. This includes your stomach, small intestine, large intestine, and rectum. A GI evaluation is an imaging test that is used to view your GI tract. This test may be used in certain cases to check for signs of cancer spread.

This imaging test uses a scope to see inside your GI tract. A scope is a long, thin tube that can be guided into your body, often through the mouth, anus, or a surgical cut. One end of the scope has a small light and camera lens to see inside your body. At the other end of the scope is an eyepiece that your doctor looks through to see the pictures shown by the camera.

2 Testing for ovarian cancer | Blood tests

Blood tests

Doctors test blood to look for signs of disease and assess your general health. These tests are not used to confirm (diagnose) ovarian cancer. But, abnormal results may signal there's a problem with certain organs or body systems.

Abnormal results may be caused by ovarian cancer or other health conditions. Blood tests are given along with other initial tests to assess for ovarian cancer. These tests may be repeated to check how well cancer treatment is working and to check for side effects.

For a blood test, your doctor will insert a needle into your vein to remove a sample of blood. Blood is often removed from a vein in the arm. The needle may bruise your skin and you may feel dizzy afterward. The blood sample will then be sent to a lab for testing. The types of blood tests used for ovarian cancer are described next.

CBC (complete blood count)
A CBC measures the number of red blood cells, white blood cells, and platelets. Your doctor will want to know if you have enough red blood cells to carry oxygen throughout your body, white blood cells to fight infections, and platelets to control bleeding. Your blood counts may be abnormal—too low or too high—because of cancer or another health problem.

Blood chemistry profile
A blood chemistry profile measures the levels of different chemicals in your blood. Chemicals in your blood come from your liver, bones, and other organs and tissues. Doctors use this test to assess the health of organs such as your liver and kidneys.

For example, doctors can test your total serum protein levels during a blood chemistry profile. This total serum protein level (measures albumin and globulin) will help your doctors learn more about your long-term nutritional status. He or she will want to know if your body is getting enough nutrients from food.

Abnormal blood chemistry levels—too high or too low—may be a sign that an organ isn't working well. Abnormal levels may also be caused by the spread of cancer or by other diseases. Thus, your doctor will consider your health and look at the whole profile when it comes to blood test results.

Liver function tests
The liver is an organ that does many important jobs, such as remove toxins from your blood. Liver function tests measure chemicals that are made or processed by the liver. Levels that are too high or low may be a sign of liver damage or cancer spread. Liver function tests are often done along with a blood chemistry profile.

CA-125 and other tumor markers
A tumor marker is a substance found in body tissue or fluid that may be a sign of cancer. CA-125 is a tumor marker for ovarian cancer. It is a protein with sugar molecules attached to it that is made by normal cells and ovarian cancer cells. High levels of CA-125 in the blood may be a sign of ovarian cancer or another health condition.

A CA-125 test measures the amount of CA-125 in the blood. This test is not used alone to diagnose ovarian cancer. But, it may be done along with other initial tests if your doctor suspects ovarian cancer. It may also be done during and after treatment to check treatment results.

2 Testing for ovarian cancer | Tissue tests | Review

Tissue tests

Biopsy

To confirm if you have ovarian cancer, a sample of tissue must be removed from your body for testing. This is called a biopsy. Doctors test tumor tissue to check for cancer cells and to look at the features of the cancer cells. Most often, the biopsy is done during treatment with surgery to remove ovarian cancer. (For surgery details, see *Surgical staging* in Part 3 and *Surgery* in Part 4.)

However, a biopsy may be done before treatment in certain, rare cases. This may be done if the cancer has spread too much to be removed by initial surgery. In such cases, an FNA (**f**ine-**n**eedle **a**spiration) biopsy or paracentesis may be used. An FNA biopsy uses a very thin needle to remove a small sample of tissue from the tumor. For paracentesis, a long, thin needle is inserted through the skin of the belly (abdomen) to remove a sample of fluid.

The biopsy samples will be sent to a pathologist for testing. A pathologist is a doctor who's an expert in testing cells to find disease. The pathologist will view the samples with a microscope to look for cancer cells. He or she will also assess the features of the cancer cells.

Review of tumor tissue

Sometimes ovarian cancer is confirmed by a prior surgery or biopsy performed by another doctor. In this case, your cancer doctors will need to review all of the prior results. This includes results of the surgery, biopsy, and tests of tissue that was removed. A pathologist will examine the tumor tissue with a microscope to make sure it is ovarian cancer. Your doctors will also want to know if the surgery left any cancer in your body. All of this will help your current doctors plan treatment done during and after treatment to check treatment results.

Review

▸ Cancer tests are used to plan treatment.

▸ Your medical and family history help inform your doctor about your health.

▸ Genetic counseling may help you decide whether to be tested for hereditary ovarian cancer.

▸ A pelvic exam checks the health of your ovaries and uterus.

▸ Imaging tests can show if there is a tumor in your ovaries and if the cancer has spread.

▸ Blood tests check for signs of disease.

▸ A biopsy is the removal of samples of tissue to test for cancer cells.

What to do...

✓ Keep a list of contact information of all of your health care providers.

✓ Keep a list of all of your current medications and supplements.

✓ Use a calendar or day planner to keep track of your appointments.

3 Cancer staging

23 Surgical staging

25 Staging systems

25 Ovarian cancer stages

30 Cancer grades and cell types

30 Cancer care plan

32 Review

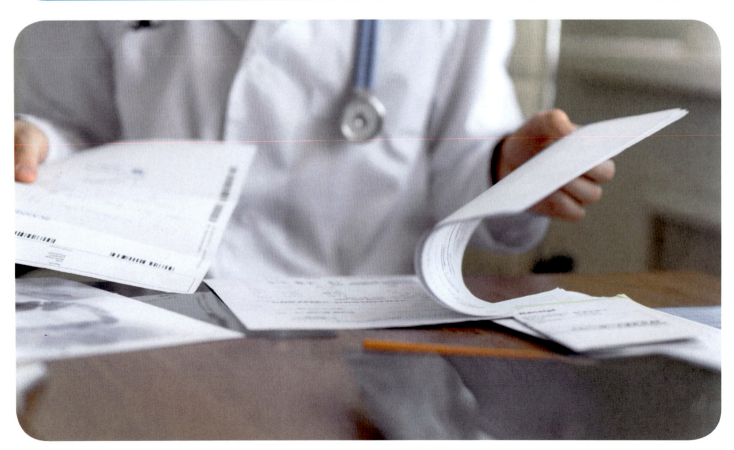

3 Cancer staging | Surgical staging

Cancer staging is the process of finding out how far the cancer has grown and spread in your body. The cancer stage is a rating of the extent of the cancer. Doctors use cancer staging to plan which treatments are best for you. Part 3 describes the staging process and defines the stages of ovarian cancer.

Surgical staging

Cancer is often staged twice. The clinical stage is based on tests done before surgery. It can give your doctors an idea of how far the cancer may have spread. But, to know the true extent of ovarian cancer, surgery is needed. The pathologic stage is based on the results of surgery and tests of tissue removed during surgery. It is the most important stage and is used to plan treatment.

During surgery to remove the cancer, your doctor will perform a number of tests to find out exactly how far it has spread. This is called surgical staging. It is the most complete and accurate way to stage ovarian cancer.

During surgical staging, your doctor will carefully inspect tissues and organs near the tumor to see where the cancer has spread.

Some tissues will be removed so they can be tested for cancer cells. This includes removing some or all of the omentum and nearby lymph nodes.

› Surgery to remove the omentum is called an **omentectomy.**

› Surgery to remove nearby lymph nodes is called a **lymph node dissection.**

Which surgical staging procedures you will have depends on how far your doctors think the cancer has spread.

Your doctor will also take biopsy samples from nearby tissues where it looks like the cancer hasn't spread. This is done to check for cancer cells that have spread but can only be seen with a microscope. These are called microscopic metastases. Your doctor will take samples from places where ovarian cancer often spreads. **See Figure 7** on the next page.

What to know...

✓ NCCN experts recommend that surgical staging be done by a gynecologic oncologist.

✓ A gynecologic oncologist is a surgeon who's an expert in cancers that start in a woman's reproductive organs.

3 Cancer staging | Surgical staging

The number of samples taken depends on how far your doctor thinks the cancer has spread. Biopsy sites may include the following:

- **Nearby lymph nodes** – groups of special disease-fighting cells

- **Pelvis** – the area below the belly (abdomen) between the hip bones

- **Abdomen** – the belly area between the chest and pelvis

- **Diaphragm** – the muscles below the ribs that help a person breathe

- **Omentum** – the layer of fatty tissue covering organs in the abdomen

- **Peritoneum** – the tissue that lines the inside of the abdomen and pelvis and covers most organs in this space

- **Ascites** – abnormal fluid buildup in the abdomen

If you don't have ascites, your doctor may "wash" the space inside your belly (peritoneal cavity) with a special liquid. This is called a peritoneal washing. Samples of the liquid will then be tested for cancer cells. These samples are called peritoneal washings, but are often referred to as "washings."

Figure 7
Possible biopsy sites in the abdomen and pelvis

Surgery is used for ovarian cancer staging. Biopsy samples will be taken from the tumor as well as other organs and tissues near the ovaries. This may include the diaphragm, omentum, peritoneum, ascites, and nearby lymph nodes.

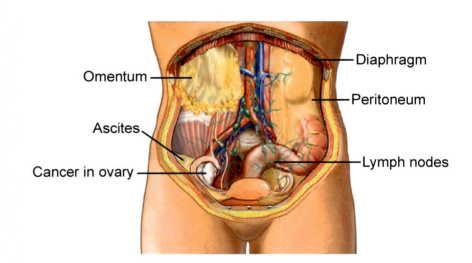

Illustration Copyright © 2017 Nucleus Medical Media, All rights reserved. www.nucleusinc.com

3 Cancer staging | Staging systems | Ovarian cancer stages

Staging systems

A staging system is a standard way to describe the extent of cancer in the body. There are two staging systems for ovarian cancer: the AJCC (**A**merican **J**oint **C**ommittee on **C**ancer) staging system and the FIGO (International **F**ederation of **G**ynecology and **O**bstetrics) staging system. These staging systems are very similar. But, the FIGO system is used most often.

In the FIGO system, the cancer stage is defined by three main areas of cancer growth:

- The extent of the first (primary) tumor
- The spread of cancer to nearby lymph nodes
- The spread of cancer to distant sites

The ovarian cancer stages are labeled by Roman numerals I, II, III, and IV. The stages are also divided into smaller groups. This helps to describe the extent of cancer in more detail. The smaller groups are labeled by adding letters and numbers to the Roman numerals. The next section describes each cancer stage as defined by the FIGO staging system.

Ovarian cancer stages

Ovarian cancers of the same stage tend to have a similar prognosis. A prognosis is the likely or expected course and outcome of a disease. In general, earlier cancer stages have better outcomes. But, doctors define cancer stages with information from thousands of patients, so a cancer stage gives an average outcome. It may not tell the outcome for one person. Some people will do better than expected. Others will do worse. Other factors not used for cancer staging, such as your general health, are also very important.

The stages of ovarian cancer are described next. The cancer stages are defined by the FIGO staging system.

The best advice that I could offer someone facing an illness is to stay positive no matter how much it tears you down, fight for the life you deserve, and please be pro-active because no one at any age, class, or race is invincible to cancer, disease, and illness.

- Christa

NCCN Guidelines for Patients®:
Ovarian Cancer, Version 1.2017

3 Cancer staging | Ovarian cancer stages

Stage I
The tumor (cancer) is only in the ovaries. Cancer may be found in one or both ovaries. But, it has not spread to any other organs or tissues in the body. **See Figure 8.**

Stage IA – Cancer is only in one ovary and the tumor is contained inside the ovary. The outer sac (capsule) of the ovary is intact. There is no cancer on the outside surface of the ovary. No cancer cells are found in ascites or washings.

Stage IB – Cancer is in both ovaries. The capsules are intact and there is no cancer on the outside surface of the ovaries. No cancer cells are found in ascites or washings.

Stage IC – Cancer is in one or both ovaries. And, one or more of the following has happened:

> **Stage IC1** – The capsule of the ovary broke open (ruptured) during surgery. This is called surgical spill.

> **Stage IC2** – The capsule ruptured before surgery, or cancer is on the outer surface of the ovary.

> **Stage IC3** – Cancer cells are found in ascites or washings.

Stage II
Cancer is in one or both ovaries and it has spread to other organs or tissues within the pelvis. Cancer has not spread outside the pelvis or to any lymph nodes. **See Figure 9.**

Stage IIA – Cancer has grown into and/or spread implants on the uterus, fallopian tubes, or both.

Stage IIB – Cancer has grown into and/or spread implants on other organs or tissues in the pelvis. This may include the bladder, sigmoid colon, rectum, or the peritoneum within the pelvis. The peritoneum is the tissue that lines the inside of the abdomen and pelvis and covers most organs in this space.

3 Cancer staging | Ovarian cancer stages

Figure 8
Stage I ovarian cancer

Stage I ovarian cancer is when cancer is only in the ovaries and has not spread to other organs.

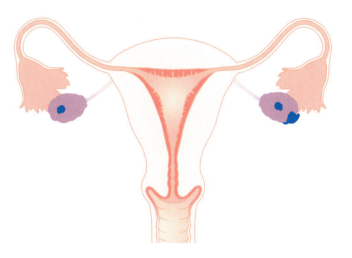

By Cancer Research UK (Original email from CRUK) [CC BY-SA 4.0 (http://creativecommons.org/licenses/by-sa/4.0)], via Wikimedia Commons

Figure 9
Stage II ovarian cancer

Stage II ovarian cancer is when the cancer has spread to other organs or tissues in the pelvis.

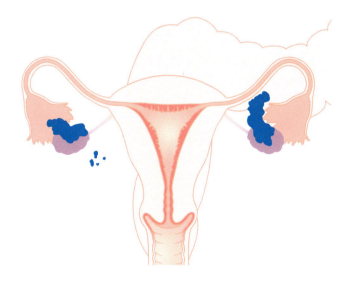

By Cancer Research UK (Original email from CRUK) [CC BY-SA 4.0 (http://creativecommons.org/licenses/by-sa/4.0)], via Wikimedia Commons

3 Cancer staging | Ovarian cancer stages

Stage III

Cancer in is one or both ovaries. It has spread outside the pelvis to tissues in the belly (abdomen). And, one or both of the following has happened: 1) cancer has spread to the tissue lining the inside of the abdomen (peritoneum); or 2) cancer may have spread to lymph nodes in the back part of the abdomen behind the peritoneum. **See Figure 10.**

Stage IIIA1 – Cancer has spread outside the pelvis, but only to lymph nodes in the back part of the abdomen—called retroperitoneal lymph nodes.

> **Stage IIIA1 (i)** – Cancer in the lymph nodes is 10 mm (millimeters) or smaller.

> **Stage IIIA1 (ii)** – Cancer in the lymph nodes is larger than 10 mm.

Stage IIIA2 – Cancer has spread to the tissue lining the abdomen, but it is so small it can only be seen with a microscope. Cancer may have also spread to lymph nodes in the back of the abdomen.

Stage IIIB – Cancer has spread to the tissue lining the abdomen and it can be seen without a microscope. The areas of cancer spread are 2 cm (centimeters) or smaller. Cancer may have also spread to lymph nodes in the back of the abdomen.

Stage IIIC – Cancer has spread to the tissue lining the abdomen and it can be seen without a microscope. The areas of cancer spread are larger than 2 cm. Cancer may have spread to lymph nodes in the back of the abdomen. It may have also spread to the outer surface of the liver or spleen.

Stage IV

Cancer has spread to distant sites in the body beyond the pelvis and abdomen. Cancer may have spread to distant organs such as the lungs, brain, or skin. It may have spread to the inside of the liver or spleen. Cancer may have also spread to lymph nodes outside the abdomen—called distant lymph nodes. **See Figure 11.**

Stage IVA – Cancer cells are found in the fluid around the lungs—called pleural effusion. But, cancer has not spread anywhere else outside the abdomen.

Stage IVB – Cancer has spread to the inside of the liver or spleen, to distant lymph nodes, or to other organs outside the abdomen.

3 Cancer staging | Ovarian cancer stages

**Figure 10
Stage III ovarian cancer**

Stage III ovarian cancer is when the cancer has spread outside the pelvis to organs or tissues in the abdomen.

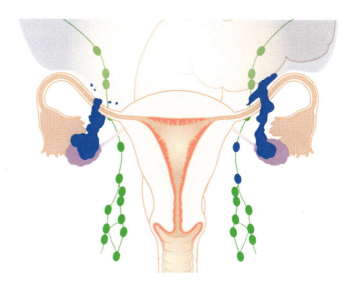

By Cancer Research UK (Original email from CRUK) [CC BY-SA 4.0 (http://creativecommons.org/licenses/by-sa/4.0)], via Wikimedia Commons

**Figure 11
Stage IV ovarian cancer**

Stage IV ovarian cancer is when the cancer has spread outside the pelvis and abdomen to organs or tissues far away in the body.

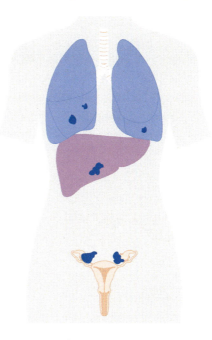

By Cancer Research UK (Original email from CRUK) [CC BY-SA 4.0 (http://creativecommons.org/licenses/by-sa/4.0)], via Wikimedia Commons

Cancer grades and cell subtypes

Ovarian cancer is also classified based on what the cancer cells look like when viewed with a microscope. A pathologist will examine the cancer cells to find out the cancer grade and cell subtype. A pathologist is a doctor who's an expert in testing cells with a microscope to identify disease. Testing cancer cells from tissue removed during surgery is the only way to find out the cancer grade and cell subtype.

Cancer grades

The cancer grade is a rating of how much the cancer cells look like normal cells. The cancer grade is a sign of how fast the cancer will likely grow and spread. Based on the features of the cancer cells, the pathologist will score the cancer as Grade 1, 2, or 3.

- **Grade 1** cancer cells look similar to normal cells. This is also called low grade. These cancer cells grow slowly and are less likely to spread.

- **Grade 2** cancer cells look more abnormal than Grade 1, but not as abnormal as Grade 3. These cancer cells grow at a medium speed. They are more likely to spread than Grade 1, but less likely than Grade 3.

- **Grade 3** cancer cells look very different from normal cells. This is also called high grade. These cancer cells grow faster and are the most likely to spread.

Some pathologists describe the grading in only two classes: high grade or low grade. Low grade includes the Grade 1 definition above. High grade includes the Grade 2 and Grade 3 definitions.

Ovarian cancer cell subtypes

Ovarian cancer is divided (classified) into smaller groups called cell subtypes. The cell subtype is based on the features of the cancer cells. A pathologist will view the cancer cells with a microscope to find out the cell subtype. There are four main cell subtypes of ovarian cancer. Serous is the most common. The other main cell subtypes are mucinous, endometrioid, and clear cell. However, all four subtypes are often treated in the same way.

Cancer care plan

Your treatment team

Treating ovarian cancer takes a team approach. Gynecologic oncologists and medical oncologists often work closely together to plan the best treatment for ovarian cancer. A gynecologic oncologist is a doctor who's an expert in surgery to treat cancers that start in a woman's reproductive organs. A medical oncologist is a doctor who is an expert in treating cancer with chemotherapy and other drugs. NCCN experts recommend that a gynecologic oncologist should perform the initial surgery for ovarian cancer when possible.

Your primary care doctor can also be part of your team. He or she can help you express your feelings about treatments to the team. Treatment of other medical problems may be improved if he or she is informed of your cancer care. Besides doctors, you may receive care from nurses, social workers, and other health experts. Ask to have the names and contact information of your health care providers included in the treatment plan.

Cancer treatment

There is no single treatment practice that is best for all patients. There is often more than one treatment option, including clinical trials. Clinical trials study how well a treatment works and its safety.

| 3 Cancer staging | Cancer care plan |

A guide to ovarian cancer treatment options can be found in Parts 5 and 6. The treatment that you and your doctors agree on should be reported in the treatment plan. It is also important to note the goal of treatment and the chance of a good treatment outcome. All known side effects should be listed and the time required to treat them should be noted. See Part 4 for a list of some common side effects of ovarian cancer treatments.

Your treatment plan may change because of new information. You may change your mind about treatment. Tests may find new results. How well the treatment is working may change. Any of these changes may require a new treatment plan.

Stress and symptom control

Cancer and its treatments can cause bothersome symptoms. The stress of having cancer can also cause symptoms. There are ways to treat many symptoms, so tell your treatment team about any that you have.

You may lose sleep before, during, and after treatment. Getting less sleep can affect your mood, conversations, and ability to do daily tasks. If possible, allow yourself to rest, let people do things for you, and talk with your doctor about sleep medication. Behavioral sleep medicine—a type of talk therapy—may also help.

Feelings of anxiety and depression are common among people with cancer. At your cancer center, cancer navigators, social workers, and other experts can help. Help can include support groups, talk therapy, or medication. Some people also feel better by exercising, talking with loved ones, or relaxing.

You may be unemployed or miss work during treatment. Or, you may have too little or no health insurance. Talk to your treatment team about work, insurance, or money problems.

They will include information in the treatment plan to help you manage your finances and medical costs.

Survivorship care

Cancer survivorship begins on the day you learn of having ovarian cancer. For many survivors, the end of active treatment signals a time of celebration but also of great anxiety. This is a very normal response. You may need support to address issues that arise from not having regular visits with your cancer care team. In addition, your treatment plan should include a schedule of follow-up cancer tests, treatment of long-term side effects, and care of your general health.

Advance care planning

Talking with your doctor about your prognosis can help with treatment planning. If the cancer can't be controlled or cured, a care plan for the end of life can be made. However, such talks often happen too late or not at all. Your doctor may delay these talks for fear that you may lose hope, become depressed, or have a shorter survival. Studies suggest that these fears are wrong. Instead, there are many benefits to advance care planning. It is useful for:

› Knowing what to expect

› Making the most of your time

› Lowering the stress of caregivers

› Having your wishes followed

› Having a better quality of life

› Getting good care

3 Cancer staging | Review

Advance care planning starts with an honest talk between you and your doctors. You don't have to know the exact details of your prognosis. Just having a general idea will help with planning. With this information, you can decide at what point you'd want to stop chemotherapy or other treatments, if at all. You can also decide what treatments you'd want for symptom relief, such as surgery or medicine.

Another part of the planning involves hospice care. Hospice care doesn't include treatment to fight the cancer but rather to reduce symptoms caused by cancer. Hospice care may be started because you aren't interested in more cancer treatment, no other cancer treatment is available, or because you may be too sick for cancer treatment.

Hospice care allows you to have the best quality of life possible. Care is given all day, every day of the week. You can choose to have hospice care at home or at a hospice center. One study found that patients and caregivers had a better quality of life when hospice care was started early.

An advance directive describes the treatment you'd want if you weren't able to make your wishes known. It also can name a person you'd want to make decisions for you. It is a legal paper that your doctors have to follow. It can reveal your wishes about life-sustaining machines, such as feeding tubes. It can also include your treatment wishes if your heart or lungs were to stop working. If you already have an advance directive, it may need to be updated to be legally valid.

Review

- Cancer staging is how doctors rate and describe the extent of cancer in the body.

- The cancer stage is a rating of how much the cancer has grown and spread.

- Ovarian cancer is grouped into stages to help plan treatment.

- Ovarian cancer is staged during surgery to remove the cancer—called surgical staging.

- The cancer grade is a rating of how much the cancer cells look like normal cells.

- The cancer grade describes how fast or slow the cancer will likely grow and spread.

- Treating ovarian cancer takes a team approach. Gynecologic oncologists and medical oncologists often work closely together to plan the best treatment for ovarian cancer.

- Your treatment plan should include a schedule of follow-up cancer tests, treatment of long-term side effects, and care of your general health.

3 Cancer staging

Ovarian cancer changed my life by causing me to slow down and enjoy every moment in life. As a survivor friend told me when I was first diagnosed, 'Of course it goes without saying that your life has changed forever, but not necessarily the way you think. There are just as many beautiful aspects to this as there are scary ones.' So look for the beauty in each and every day because it is there and it will give you the strength to keep going.

- Alicia

4 Overview of cancer treatments

35 Surgery

37 Chemotherapy

39 Targeted therapy

40 Hormone therapy

41 Clinical trials

42 Review

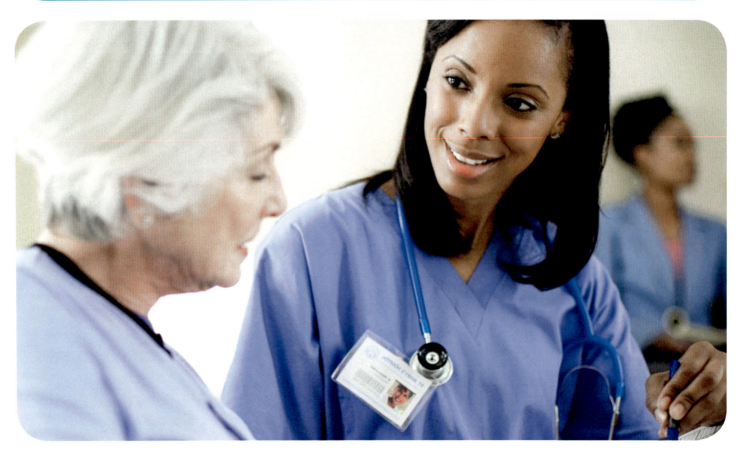

4 Cancer treatments | Surgery

Part 4 describes the main types of treatment for ovarian cancer. This information may help you understand the treatment options listed in the Treatment guide in Parts 5 and 6. It may also help you know what to expect during treatment. Not every person with ovarian cancer will receive every treatment listed.

Surgery

Surgery is used as the first and main (primary) treatment for most ovarian cancers. Primary treatment is the main treatment given to rid the body of cancer. NCCN experts recommend that ovarian cancer surgery should be performed by a gynecologic oncologist. A gynecologic oncologist is a surgeon who is an expert in cancers that start in a woman's reproductive organs. Gynecologic oncologists and medical oncologists often work closely together to plan the best treatment for ovarian cancer. A medical oncologist is a doctor who is an expert in treating cancer with chemotherapy and other drugs.

There are two main goals of surgical treatment for ovarian cancer. One goal is to find out how far the cancer has spread. The other goal of surgery is to remove all or as much of the cancer from your body as possible. To do so, the tumor is removed along with other organs and tissues where cancer cells have or might have spread.

A number of procedures may be done during surgical treatment for ovarian cancer. The type and extent of surgery you will have depends on many factors. This includes the tumor size, tumor location, and how far the cancer has spread. Another key factor is whether or not you want to be able to have babies after treatment.

Types of surgical treatment

Surgical treatment often involves removing both ovaries, both fallopian tubes, and the uterus.

- A **BSO (bilateral salpingo-oophorectomy)** is surgery to remove both ovaries and both fallopian tubes.

- A **USO (unilateral salpingo-oophorectomy)** is surgery to remove only one ovary and the attached fallopian tube.

A USO is also called "fertility-sparing surgery." This is because you will still be able to have babies after the surgery if you haven't yet gone through menopause. A USO is only an option if the cancer is only in one ovary.

A hysterectomy is surgery to remove the uterus. When the uterus and the cervix are removed, it is called a total hysterectomy. Most often, the uterus and cervix are removed through a surgical cut in the belly (abdomen). This is called a TAH (**t**otal **a**bdominal **h**ysterectomy) and it is done along with a BSO. You will not be able to have babies after a TAH and BSO.

If cancer has spread outside the ovaries, then your doctor will try to remove as much of the cancer as possible. This is called debulking surgery or cytoreductive surgery. During this surgery, your doctor will attempt to remove all of the cancer that can be seen. If the surgeon is able to remove all of the tumors that are 1 cm or larger in size, the surgery is called an optimal debulking. Optimal debulking is linked with better treatment outcomes.

4 Cancer treatments | Surgery

Debulking surgery may remove all or part of nearby organs where cancer has spread. **See Figure 12.** This may include removing organs such as your spleen, gallbladder, and appendix. It may also remove part of your stomach, liver, pancreas, bladder, diaphragm, and intestines. Lymph nodes that look different or are larger than normal should also be removed if possible.

Surgery methods

Most often, surgery is done using a laparotomy. A laparotomy is a long surgical cut in the abdomen. It is often an up-and-down (vertical) cut from the top of the belly button down to the pelvic bone. This lets your doctor see the tumor and other organs and tissues in your abdomen and pelvis.

Thus, a laparotomy is the most common and preferred method for ovarian cancer surgery. NCCN experts recommend that it should be used when surgical staging or debulking surgery is planned.

Laparoscopy is another surgery method that may be used in some cases. Laparoscopy uses a few small cuts in the abdomen instead of one big one. Small tools are inserted through the cuts to perform the surgery. One of the tools is called a laparoscope. It is a long tube with a light and camera at the end. The camera lets your doctor see your ovaries and other tissues inside your abdomen. The other tools are used to remove tissue.

Figure 12
Debulking surgery sites

Debulking surgery removes as much cancer as possible. The extent of the surgery depends on how far the cancer has spread. It may remove all or part of nearby organs such as your liver, spleen, stomach, gallbladder, pancreas, intestines, appendix, and bladder.

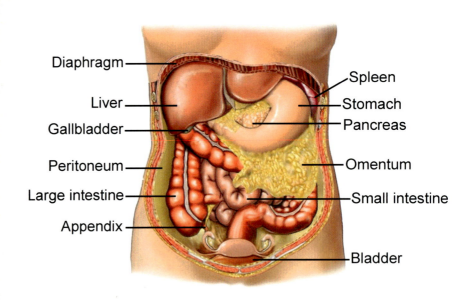

Illustration Copyright © 2017 Nucleus Medical Media, All rights reserved. www.nucleusinc.com

| 4 Cancer treatments | Chemotherapy |

Laparoscopy may be used in select cases, such as when cancer is only in the ovaries. Rarely, it may be used when cancer has spread outside the ovaries. This surgery should only be done by a gynecologic oncologist with a lot of experience.

Preparing for surgery

Your treatment team will give you instructions on how to prepare for your surgery. You may be asked to stop taking some medicines for a short time. You also should not eat or drink after midnight the night before the surgery.

On the day of your surgery, you will be given medicine to put you into a deep sleep so you won't feel pain. This is called general anesthesia. Surgery may take three or more hours to complete. More or less time may be needed depending on how much tissue is removed.

After the surgery, you will need to stay in the hospital for a few days or weeks to recover. You may feel some pain and tenderness in your belly and pelvis. This may last for a few days or weeks. You may not be able to return to normal activities in a few weeks. The time it takes to fully recover varies from person to person. It also varies depending on the extent of the surgery.

Risks and side effects of surgery

With any type of surgery, there are some health risks and side effects. A side effect is an unhealthy or unpleasant condition caused by treatment. Common side effects of any surgery include pain, swelling, and scars. But, the side effects of surgery can differ between people. They also differ based on the type and extent of surgery.

Some common side effects of surgery for ovarian cancer include leg swelling, trouble urinating, and constipation. If you haven't gone through menopause, then surgery that removes both ovaries will cause menopause.

Menopause is the point in time when you won't have another menstrual period again. When caused by surgery, the symptoms of menopause may be sudden and more severe. Symptoms of menopause include hot flashes, changes in mood, trouble sleeping, vaginal dryness, weight gain, and night sweats.

All of the side effects of ovarian cancer surgery are not listed here. Ask your treatment team for a full list of common and rare side effects. If a side effect bothers you, tell your treatment team. There may be ways to help you feel better.

Chemotherapy

Chemotherapy is the use of drugs to kill cancer cells. Many people refer to this treatment as "chemo." Chemotherapy drugs kill fast-growing cells throughout the body, including cancer cells and normal cells.

Most women with ovarian cancer receive chemotherapy after primary treatment with surgery. This is called adjuvant treatment. Your doctor may also refer to this as primary chemotherapy. In certain cases, chemotherapy may be given to shrink the cancer before surgery.

Different types of chemotherapy drugs attack cancer cells in different ways. Some kill cancer cells by damaging their DNA (**d**eoxyribo**n**ucleic **a**cid)— molecules that contain coded instructions for making and controlling cells. Others interfere with parts of cells that are needed for making new cells.

Many types of chemotherapy drugs are used for ovarian cancer. Two of the main types used are platinum agents and taxanes. Platinum agents damage DNA in cells, which stops them from making new cells and causes them to die.

4 Cancer treatments | Chemotherapy

Some platinum agents used for ovarian cancer are carboplatin, cisplatin, and oxaliplatin.

Taxanes block certain cell parts to stop a cell from dividing into two cells. Some taxanes used for ovarian cancer are paclitaxel, paclitaxel albumin-bound, and docetaxel. Guide 2 lists the chemotherapy drugs that are used for ovarian cancer.

Guide 2. Chemotherapy drugs

Generic name	Brand name (sold as)
Altretamine	Hexalen®
Capecitabine	Xeloda®
Carboplatin	--
Cisplatin	Platinol®
Cyclophosphamide	--
Docetaxel	Taxotere®
Doxorubicin	Adriamycin®
Doxorubicin, liposome injection	Doxil®
Etoposide, oral	--
Gemcitabine	Gemzar®
Ifosfamide	--
Irinotecan	Camptosar®
Melphalan	Alkeran®
Oxaliplatin	Eloxatin®
Paclitaxel	Taxol®
Paclitaxel, albumin-bound	Abraxane®
Pemetrexed	Alimta®
Topotecan	Hycamtin®
Vinorelbine	Navelbine

Because chemotherapy drugs differ in how they work, more than one drug is often used. A combination regimen is the use of two or more drugs. When only one drug is used, it is called a single agent. A regimen is a treatment plan that specifies the drug(s), dose, schedule, and length of treatment. The most common regimens used for initial chemotherapy treatment are:

› Paclitaxel and carboplatin

› Paclitaxel and carboplatin (weekly)

› Dose-dense paclitaxel and carboplatin

› Paclitaxel and cisplatin

› Docetaxel and carboplatin

Chemotherapy is given in cycles. A cycle includes days of treatment followed by days of rest. Giving chemotherapy in cycles lets the body have a chance to recover before the next treatment. The cycles vary in length depending on which drugs are used. Often, the cycles are 7, 14, 21, or 28 days long. The number of treatment days per cycle and the number of cycles given also varies depending on the regimen used.

How chemotherapy is given
Most of the chemotherapy drugs for ovarian cancer are liquids that are slowly injected into a vein. This is called an IV (intravenous) infusion. Some drugs, such as etoposide and altretamine, are pills that are swallowed.

Chemotherapy can also be given as a liquid that is slowly injected into the abdomen (peritoneal cavity). This is called IP (intraperitoneal) chemotherapy. When given this way, higher doses of the drugs are delivered directly to the cancer cells in the belly area.

4 Cancer treatments | Targeted therapy

IP chemotherapy is given through a thin tube called a catheter. The catheter is often placed inside the abdomen during surgery. Studies have shown that patients live longer when they are able to receive some of their chemotherapy in this manner.

Side effects of chemotherapy

A side effect is an unhealthy or unpleasant physical or emotional condition caused by treatment. Each treatment for ovarian cancer can cause side effects. How your body will respond can't be fully known. Some people have many side effects. Others have few. Some side effects can be very serious while others can be unpleasant but not serious.

The side effects of chemotherapy depend on many factors. This includes the drug, the dose, and the person. In general, side effects are caused by the death of fast-growing cells, which are found in the intestines, mouth, and blood. As a result, common side effects include not feeling hungry, nausea, vomiting, mouth sores, hair loss, fatigue, low blood cell counts, increased risk of infection, bleeding or bruising easily, and nerve damage (neuropathy).

Some side effects are more likely or more severe when certain combination regimens are used. The docetaxel and carboplatin regimen is more likely to increase the risk of infection. The paclitaxel and carboplatin regimen is more likely to cause neuropathy. Neuropathy is a nerve problem that causes pain, tingling, and numbness in the hands and feet. Side effects also differ depending on how chemotherapy is given. IP chemotherapy tends to cause more severe side effects than IV chemotherapy. This includes infections, kidney damage, pain in the belly, and nerve damage.

Not all side effects of chemotherapy are listed here. Be sure to ask your treatment team for a full list of common and rare side effects of the drugs you receive.

If a side effect bothers you, tell your treatment team. There may be ways to help you feel better.

Targeted therapy

Targeted therapy is treatment with drugs that target a specific or unique feature of cancer cells. These drugs stop the action of molecules that help cancer cells grow. Targeted therapy is less likely to harm normal cells than chemotherapy. Some targeted therapy drugs that are approved to treat ovarian cancer are bevacizumab (Avastin®), olaparib (Lynparza®) and rucaparib (Rubraca™), and niraparib (Zejula®). Pazopanib (Votrient®) is another targeted therapy drug that is sometimes used for ovarian cancer. These drugs attack cancer cells in different ways.

Bevacizumab

Bevacizumab is a type of targeted therapy called an angiogenesis inhibitor. Angiogenesis is the growth of new blood vessels. Like normal cells, cancer cells need the food and oxygen delivered in blood to live and grow. Cancer cells send out signals that cause new blood vessels to grow into the tumor to "feed" it. Bevacizumab blocks these signals so that new blood vessels will not form. As a result, the cancer cells won't receive the blood they need to live.

Some common side effects of bevacizumab are high blood pressure, headache, nosebleeds, runny nose, taste changes, skin rash, dry skin, and back pain. Rare but serious side effects include stroke, heart attack, kidney damage, holes in the intestine, and bleeding within the body.

Olaparib, rucaparib, and niraparib

Olaparib, rucaparib, and niraparib are a type of targeted therapy known as PARP (**p**oly **A**DP-**r**ibose **p**olymerase) inhibitors. PARP is a protein that helps repair damaged DNA in cells.

4 Cancer treatments | Hormone therapy

The *BRCA1* and *BRCA2* genes also help repair DNA damage in cells. But, mutations in these genes prevent them from making needed repairs. When cancer cells have mutations in the *BRCA* genes, they now must rely on PARP to repair DNA. These drugs block the action of PARP so that the PARP can no longer repair DNA damage in any cells. This now makes it very hard for cancer cells with *BRCA* mutations to repair damaged DNA. If a cell is not able to repair damaged DNA, it will die.

While all three drugs work the same, each of these agents have been approved for certain use to treat ovarian cancer. Typically patients need to have a *BRCA1* or *BRCA2* germline mutation. For example, olaparib is used in patients with *BRCA* mutations who have progressed after three lines of prior chemotherapy treatment. Rucaparib is given to those who have recurrent disease that is platinum sensitive. Platinum sensitive means the cancer initially responded to a platinum-based chemotherapy but the cancer came back (recurred) more than 6 months after treatment. Niraparib is used in the recurrent setting but as maintenance therapy (to help maintain a good response) after a platinum-based chemotherapy.

Some common side effects of olaparib, rucaparib, and niraparib are nausea, vomiting, diarrhea, stomach pain, muscle or joint pain, feeling tired or weak, not feeling hungry, and low blood cell counts.

Pazopanib
Pazopanib is a type of targeted therapy called a TKI (**t**yrosine **k**inase **i**nhibitor). Tyrosine kinases are proteins in cells that are important for many cell functions. This includes sending signals in cells for cell growth, survival, and death.

Some tyrosine kinases send signals that tell cancer cells to grow and divide to make new cells. Some send signals for new blood vessels to grow into the tumor so it can survive. Pazopanib targets several tyrosine kinases and blocks the signals that help cancer grow and spread. Blocking these signals may slow cancer growth.

Common side effects of pazopanib include diarrhea, high blood pressure, and change in hair color, nausea, vomiting, fatigue, and not feeling hungry.

Hormone therapy

Hormone therapy is treatment that stops the body from making certain hormones or stops the action of the hormones. Hormone therapy is not used as initial treatment for ovarian cancer. But, it may be used for ovarian cancer that has come back after other treatments.

Estrogen and progesterone are hormones that help some ovarian cancers grow. Estrogen is mostly made by the ovaries and is made in small amounts by the adrenal glands, liver, and body fat. Progesterone is also mostly made by the ovaries. Blocking these hormones from working or lowering hormone levels may help slow ovarian cancer growth.

Different types of hormone therapy drugs work in different ways. The hormone therapy drugs that may be used for ovarian cancer include:

> Tamoxifen – This drug stops the effect of estrogen on cancer cell growth. It is in a class of drugs called antiestrogens.

> Anastrozole, exemestane, and letrozole – These drugs lower estrogen levels in the body. They are in a class of drugs called aromatase inhibitors.

4 Cancer treatments | Clinical trials

> Leuprolide acetate – This drug causes the ovaries to make less estrogen and progesterone. It is in a class of drugs called LHRH (luteinizing hormone-releasing hormone) agonists.

> Megestrol acetate – This drug stops the effect of estrogen on cancer cell growth. It is in a class of drugs called progestins.

Hormone therapy can cause a number of side effects. A side effect is an unhealthy or unpleasant response to treatment. The side effects may be mild or severe. Symptoms of menopause are common. Such symptoms include hot flashes, changes in mood, vaginal dryness, trouble sleeping, and night sweats. Other common side effects of hormone therapy are vaginal discharge, weight gain, swelling in the hands and feet, fatigue, and less interest in sex. Blood clots are a rare but serious side effect of tamoxifen. Aromatase inhibitors can weaken your bones and may also cause joint and muscle pain.

All of the side effects of hormone therapy are not listed here. Ask your treatment team for a full list of common and rare side effects of the drug you receive. If a side effect bothers you, tell your treatment team. There may be ways to help you feel better.

Clinical trials

A clinical trial is a type of research study that people choose to take part in as part of their cancer care. Clinical trials help doctors learn how to prevent, diagnose, and treat a disease like cancer. Because of clinical trials, doctors find safe and helpful ways to improve cancer care. This guide provides information about many of those tests and treatments used to help people with cancer.

Complementary and alternative medicine

CAM (**c**omplementary and **a**lternative **m**edicine) is a group of treatments sometimes used by people with cancer. Many CAMs are being studied to see if they are truly helpful.

> Complementary medicines are meant to be used alongside standard therapies, most often for relaxation, improving your health, or to prevent or reduce side effects.

> Alternative medicine is treatment or techniques that are used instead of standard treatments such as chemotherapy or radiation. Some are sold as cures even though they haven't been proven to work in clinical trials.

Many cancer centers or local hospitals have complementary therapy programs that offer acupuncture, yoga, and other types of therapy.

It's important to tell your treatment team if you are using any complementary medicine, especially supplements, vitamins, or herbs. Some of these things can interfere with your cancer treatment. For more information about CAM, ask your doctor and visit the websites in Part 7.

4 Cancer treatments | Review

Clinical trials go through levels or phases of testing. These phases help move the research along to find out what works best for patients with cancer.

> **Phase I** looks at how much drug to give, its side effects, and how often to give the treatment.

> **Phase II** also tests for side effects and how it works on a particular cancer type.

> **Phase III** compares the new treatment (or new use of treatment) to what is commonly used.

> **Phase IV** follows late side effects and if the treatment still works after a long period.

All clinical trials have a plan and are carefully led by a medical team. Patients in a clinical trial are often alike with their cancer type and general health. You can join a clinical trial when you meet certain terms (eligibility criteria).

If you decide to join a trial, you will need to review and sign a paper called an informed consent form. This form describes the clinical trial in detail, including the risks and benefits. Even after you sign consent, you can stop taking part in a clinical trial at any time.

Some benefits of a clinical trial:

> You'll have access to the most current cancer care

> You will be closely watched by your medical team

> You may help other patients with cancer

Some risks of a clinical trial:

> Like any test or treatment, there may be side effects

> New tests or treatments may not work

> You may have to visit the hospital more

Ask your doctor or nurse if a clinical trial may be an option for you. It is very important to keep an open mind about clinical trials and talk to your medical care team about the best option for you. There may be clinical trials available where you're getting treatment or at other treatment centers nearby. You can also find clinical trials through the websites listed in Part 7, *Resources*.

Review

> Primary treatment is the main treatment used to rid the body of cancer.

> Surgery is often used as primary treatment for ovarian cancer.

> Chemotherapy drugs kill fast-growing cells, including cancer cells and normal cells.

> Targeted therapy drugs target a specific or unique feature of cancer cells.

> Hormone therapy stops the body from making certain hormones or stops the action of the hormones.

> A clinical trial studies a test or treatment to see how safe it is and how well it works.

4 Cancer treatments

My cancer experience has been a journey of self awareness. Along the way, I have met some inspiring women who have enriched my life. As I reach my 30th year of survivorship, I realize that hope and love sustained me through those early dark days. There is no such thing as false hope; we are all entitled to hope; hope that tomorrow will be a better day. And, of course, the love of family and friends.

- Risa

5 Treatment guide for epithelial ovarian cancer

45 Stage I ovarian cancer

51 Stages II, III, and IV ovarian cancer

58 Follow-up after initial treatment

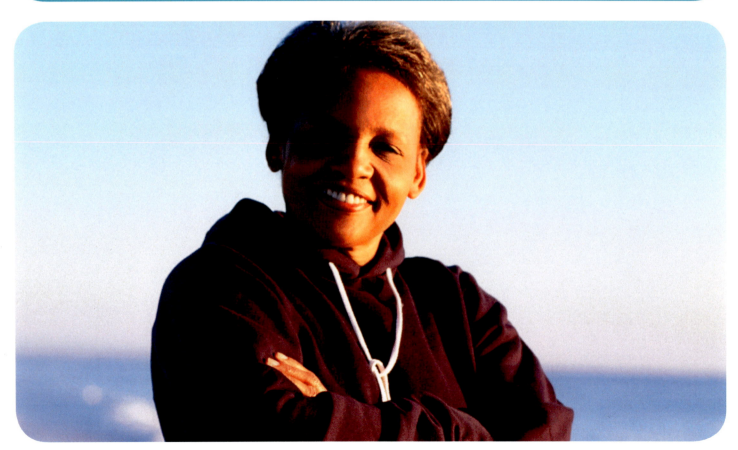

5 Treatment guide | Stage I ovarian cancer

Part 5 is a guide through the treatment options for people with epithelial ovarian cancer. It shows which tests and treatments are recommended under which conditions. This treatment information may help you ask your doctor questions about your next steps of care.

This information is taken from the treatment guidelines written by NCCN experts of ovarian cancer. These treatment guidelines list options for people with ovarian cancer in general. Thus, your doctors may suggest other treatment for you based on your health and personal needs. Discuss and decide on your treatment plan with your doctor.

Stage I ovarian cancer

Guide 3. Primary treatment for newly diagnosed ovarian cancer

Cancer stage	Treatment options
Stage IA Cancer is only in one ovary	• Surgery to remove one ovary and its fallopian tube + surgical staging + debulking as needed (fertility desired) • Surgery to remove both ovaries, both fallopian tubes, and the uterus + surgical staging
Stage IB Cancer is in both ovaries only	• Surgery to remove both ovaries and its fallopian tube + surgical staging (fertility desired) • Surgery to remove both ovaries, both fallopian tubes, and the uterus + surgical staging + debulking as needed
Stage IC Cancer is in one or both ovaries and cancer is on the ovary surface, the ovary capsule has ruptured, and/or cancer cells are in ascites or washings	• Surgery to remove one ovary and its fallopian tube + surgical staging (certain patients) • Surgery to remove both ovaries, both fallopian tubes, and the uterus + surgical staging + debulking as needed

5 Treatment guide | Stage I ovarian cancer

Guide 3 (on page 45) shows the primary treatment options for newly diagnosed stage I ovarian cancer. For ovarian cancer confirmed by a prior surgery, see Guide 4. Stage I ovarian cancer is when cancer is only in the ovaries and has not spread to other tissues or organs.

Primary treatment is the main treatment used to rid the body of cancer. Surgery is used as primary treatment for stage I ovarian cancer. Surgery is also used to find out how far the cancer has spread—called surgical staging. The type and extent of surgery you will have depends on the cancer stage and other factors. For full details on each surgery, see page 35.

Primary treatment options

The most common treatment for stage I ovarian cancer is surgery to remove both ovaries, both fallopian tubes, and the uterus. This is the only recommended option when cancer is in both ovaries—stage IB. If cancer is only in one ovary—stage IA or IC—a second option is surgery to remove the ovary with cancer and its fallopian tube. This is called fertility-sparing surgery. It may be used if you want to be able to have babies after treatment.

Along with either of these options, you will also have surgical staging. Surgical staging involves taking biopsy samples of the tumor and nearby tissues to test for cancer cells. It is done to check for cancer cells that have spread outside the ovaries or pelvis and can only be seen with a microscope. These are called microscopic metastases. During surgical staging, biopsy samples will be taken from organs and tissues where ovarian cancer often spreads. The omentum and nearby lymphs will also be removed.

Next steps

After completing primary treatment, see Guide 5 on page 49 or treatments that are recommended next.

5 Treatment guide — Stage I ovarian cancer

Guide 4. Primary treatment for ovarian cancer confirmed by prior surgery or biopsy

Results of prior surgery or biopsy	Primary treatment options
Surgery and staging complete	• No more surgery needed
Likely stage IA or IB, grade 1 Cancer is in one or both ovaries only and it is low grade (slow-growing)	• Surgical staging
Likely stage IA or IB, grade 2 Cancer is in one or both ovaries only and it is medium grade	*If doctor considers observation* • Surgical staging *If doctors think no cancer remains* • Surgical staging • Completion surgery and surgical staging • No more surgery, start chemotherapy (6 cycles) *If doctors think some cancer remains* • Completion surgery and surgical staging
Likely stage IA or IB, grade 3 or clear cell, or stage IC Cancer is in one or both ovaries only, and it's high grade (fast-growing), or cancer is also on the ovary surface, the ovary capsule has ruptured, and/or cancer cells are in ascites or washings	*If doctors think no cancer remains* • Completion surgery and surgical staging • No more surgery, start chemotherapy (6 cycles) *If doctors think some cancer remains* • Completion surgery and surgical staging

Guide 4 shows the primary treatment options for stage I ovarian cancer that was confirmed by a prior surgery or biopsy. Stage I ovarian cancer is when cancer is only in the ovaries and has not spread to other tissues or organs. Primary treatment is the main treatment used to rid the body of cancer.

Surgery is often used as primary treatment for stage I ovarian cancer. But, there is more than one option and more than one type of surgery to choose from. Which option is best for you depends on a few key factors.

The main factor is whether or not the prior surgery and staging were complete. Surgical staging is considered complete if the prior surgery removed all of the cancer, both ovaries, both fallopian tubes, the uterus, nearby supporting tissues, the omentum, and nearby lymph nodes.

The cancer stage and cancer grade are also important. The cancer stage describes how far the cancer has grown and spread. The cancer grade describes how fast the cancer will likely grow based on how much the cancer cells look like normal cells.

5 Treatment guide — Stage I ovarian cancer

Grade 1 cancer tends to grow more slowly, grade 3 tends to grow more quickly, and grade 2 is in between. See page 30 for more details about cancer grades.

Primary treatment options

To plan primary treatment, your doctor will first assess the results of the prior surgery. If the prior surgery and staging were complete, then no more surgery is needed at this time. See *Next steps* at the end of this section.

If surgery and staging were not complete, then more surgery is recommended. This is to confirm the cancer stage and, if needed, remove any remaining cancer. The type and extent of surgery depends on the likely cancer stage, cancer grade, and how much (if any) cancer remains.

For ovarian cancer that is likely stage IA or IB, grade 1, surgical staging is recommended. Surgical staging involves taking biopsy samples of the tumor and nearby tissues to test for cancer cells. It is done to check for cancer cells that have spread outside the ovaries or pelvis and can only be seen with a microscope. These are called microscopic metastases. During surgical staging, biopsy samples will be taken from organs and tissues where ovarian cancer often spreads. The omentum and nearby lymph nodes will also be removed.

For ovarian cancer that is likely stage IA or IB, grade 2, the treatment options depend on whether or not the prior surgery removed all of the cancer. If your doctor thinks no cancer remains, then you have three options to choose from. The first option is to have surgical staging alone as described above. The second option is to have completion surgery and surgical staging. Completion surgery removes the remaining ovary (or ovaries), fallopian tubes, uterus, nearby supporting tissue, the omentum, and any cancer that can be seen.

The third option is to start treatment with chemotherapy instead of having more surgery. If your doctor thinks some cancer remains, then completion surgery and surgical staging are recommended.

For ovarian cancer that is likely stage IA or IB, grade 3 or clear cell, or stage IC, the treatment options depend on whether or not the prior surgery removed all of the cancer. If your doctor thinks no cancer remains, then one option is to have completion surgery and surgical staging. Another option is to start treatment with chemotherapy instead of having more surgery. If your doctor thinks some cancer remains, then completion surgery and surgical staging are recommended.

5 Treatment guide — Stage I ovarian cancer

Guide 5. Treatment after surgery for stage I ovarian cancer

Cancer stage	Treatment options
Stage IA or IB, grade 1 Cancer is in one or both ovaries only and it is low grade (slow-growing)	• Observation with follow-up tests
Stage IA or IB, grade 2 Cancer is in one or both ovaries only and it is medium grade	• Observation with follow-up tests • Chemotherapy given in a vein (IV) for 3 to 6 cycles
Stage IA or IB, grade 3 Cancer is in one or both ovaries only, and it is high grade (fast-growing)	• Chemotherapy given in a vein (IV) for 3 to 6 cycles
Stage IC, grades 1, 2 or 3 Cancer is in one or both ovaries and cancer is on the ovary surface, the ovary capsule has ruptured, and/or cancer cells are in ascites or washings	• Chemotherapy given in a vein (IV) for 3 to 6 cycles

Chemotherapy regimens for stage I ovarian cancer

Chemotherapy regimens	Length of a cycle
Paclitaxel and carboplatin	21 days (3 weeks)
Paclitaxel and carboplatin	7 days (1 week)
Docetaxel and carboplatin	21 days (3 weeks)

5 Treatment guide — Stage I ovarian cancer

Guide 5 shows the options that are recommended after surgery for stage I ovarian cancer. Most women with ovarian cancer will receive chemotherapy after primary treatment with surgery. This is called adjuvant treatment. Your doctor may also refer to this as primary chemotherapy.

Which option is recommended after surgery depends on the cancer stage and the cancer grade. The cancer stage is a rating of how much the cancer has grown and spread. The cancer grade describes how fast the cancer will likely grow based on how much the cancer cells look like normal cells. Grade 1 cancer tends to grow more slowly, grade 3 tends to grow more quickly, and grade 2 is in between.

Treatment options

For stage IA or IB ovarian cancer, the options depend on the cancer grade. For grade 1, observation with follow-up tests is recommended. Observation is a period of testing to watch for cancer growth after treatment. For grade 2, observation with follow-up tests is still an option. A second option is to receive chemotherapy given in a vein. This is called IV chemotherapy. For all other stage I ovarian cancers, IV chemotherapy is the only recommended option.

The number of chemotherapy cycles recommended depends on whether or not surgical staging was completed. It may have been completed during the initial surgery or a second surgery. If so, 3 to 6 cycles of chemotherapy should be given. If surgical staging was not completed, then at least 6 cycles should be given.

Guide 5 also shows the chemotherapy regimens that are recommended for stage I ovarian cancer. Which drug or regimen is best for you depends on a number of factors. This includes your age, overall health, and performance status—a rating of how well you are able to do daily activities.

Another key factor is your risk for peripheral neuropathy—a nerve problem that causes pain, tingling, and numbness typically in the hands and feet.

Neuropathy is a common side effect of paclitaxel and to a less degree carboplatin. If you have a high risk for nerve problems, then docetaxel and carboplatin may be a better option for you. Some patients may not be able to tolerate the severe side effects of chemotherapy. This includes patients who are older than 65, have other health problems, or have trouble doing daily activities. For these patients, paclitaxel and carboplatin given once a week may be a good option. Giving these drugs once a week may cause fewer side effects than when they are given once every three weeks. It may be better tolerated by certain patients.

Testing during chemotherapy treatment

During treatment, your doctor will give tests to check how well the chemotherapy is working and to assess for side effects. A physical and pelvic exam may be done at least every 2 to 3 cycles. You may also have other tests as needed. This may include imaging tests, CBC, blood chemistry profile, and tests of CA-125 or other tumor markers.

Next steps

See Guide 10 on page 58 for follow-up tests that are recommended during observation and after completing chemotherapy treatment.

5 Treatment guide | Stages II, III, and IV ovarian cancer

Stages II, III, and IV ovarian cancer

Guide 6. Primary treatment for newly diagnosed ovarian cancer

Cancer stage	Primary treatment options
Stage II, III, or IV (surgery may be an option) Cancer has spread to nearby organs and tissues in the pelvis, outside the pelvis, or outside the abdomen	• Surgery to remove both ovaries, both fallopian tubes, and the uterus + surgical staging + debulking as needed
Stage III or IV (surgery may not be an option, disease is large) Cancer has spread outside the pelvis to the tissue lining the abdomen and/or to nearby lymph nodes, or cancer has spread to organs outside the abdomen	• Seek an expert opinion from a gynecologist oncologist • Biopsy to confirm type of ovarian cancer • Start chemotherapy to shrink the cancer (neoadjuvant treatment), then surgery as described above

Guide 6 shows the primary treatment options for newly diagnosed stage II, III, and IV ovarian cancer. For ovarian cancer confirmed by a prior surgery, see Guide 7. Primary treatment is the main treatment given to rid the body of cancer. The primary treatment options depend on the cancer stage. The cancer stage is a rating of how far the cancer has grown and spread.

Stage II ovarian cancer is when cancer has spread to nearby organs in the pelvis such as the other ovary, the fallopian tubes, and the uterus. Stage III ovarian cancer has spread outside the pelvis to tissues in the abdomen. Stage IV ovarian cancer has spread outside the abdomen to distant sites.

Primary treatment

Surgery is often used as primary treatment for ovarian cancer. The type and extent of surgery depends on the cancer stage. For more details about each type of surgery, see page 35.

For stage II ovarian cancer, you will have surgery to remove both ovaries, both fallopian tubes, the uterus, and all cancer that can be seen. Surgical staging procedures should also be done. This is to check for cancer cells that have spread outside the pelvis and can only be seen with a microscope. During surgical staging, biopsy samples will be taken from nearby organs and tissues where ovarian cancer often spreads. The omentum and nearby lymph nodes will also be removed.

For stage III or IV ovarian cancer, the treatment options depend on how much tissue the cancer has grown into. If the cancer hasn't grown into a lot of tissue and can be safely removed, then surgery is recommended. In this case, surgery will remove both ovaries, both fallopian tubes, the uterus, and all or as much cancer as possible. Surgery may also remove all or part of organs or tissues the cancer has spread to. This is called debulking surgery or cytoreductive surgery. It aims to reduce the amount of cancer in your body as much as possible.

5 Treatment guide | Stages II, III, and IV ovarian cancer

The goal is to not leave behind any tumors that are 1 cm or larger. Surgical staging isn't needed because the cancer has spread outside the pelvis.

If the cancer has grown into a lot of tissue, it might not be possible to safely remove it all with initial surgery. Your doctors may decide to give chemotherapy first to try to shrink the cancer before surgery. This is called preoperative or neoadjuvant chemotherapy. (See Guide 2 on page 38 for chemotherapy recommendations.) It is important that a gynecologic oncologist is involved in this assessment and treatment decision. You will likely have a biopsy (core biopsy preferred) to confirm ovarian cancer before starting chemotherapy treatment.

After a few cycles of chemotherapy, your doctor will check the status of the cancer. If your doctor thinks all the cancer can be safely removed, then you will have surgery as described above. You will likely then receive additional chemotherapy after an interval surgery.

Next steps

After primary treatment for newly diagnosed stage II, III, and IV ovarian cancer, see Guide 8 on page 54 for treatments that are recommended next.

Guide 7 shows the primary treatment options for stage II, III, and IV ovarian cancers confirmed by a prior surgery or biopsy. The cancer stage is a rating of how far the cancer has grown and spread.

Stage II ovarian cancer is when cancer has spread to nearby organs in the pelvis such as the other ovary, the fallopian tubes, and the uterus. Stage III ovarian cancer has spread outside the pelvis to tissues in the abdomen. Stage IV ovarian cancer has spread outside the abdomen to distant sites.

Surgery is often used as primary treatment for ovarian cancer. But, there is more than one option and more than one type of surgery to choose from. Which option is best for you depends on a few key factors.

If the remaining cancer can likely be removed, then tumor reductive surgery is recommended. Your doctor will remove as much as the cancer as he or she possibly can. This is called tumor reduction or a "debulking" procedure.

If all the remaining cancer likely can't be removed, then chemotherapy may be given in a vein to try to shrink the cancer before surgery. This is called neoadjuvant treatment. After a few cycles of chemotherapy, your doctors will check the status of the cancer. If your doctors think all the cancer can be safely removed, then you will have completion surgery as described above. Completion surgery after 3 cycles of chemotherapy is preferred. But, surgery may be performed after 4 to 6 cycles based on your doctor's judgment.

NCCN Guidelines for Patients®:
Ovarian Cancer, Version 1.2017

5 Treatment guide — Stages II, III, and IV ovarian cancer

Guide 7. Primary treatment for ovarian cancer confirmed by prior surgery or biopsy

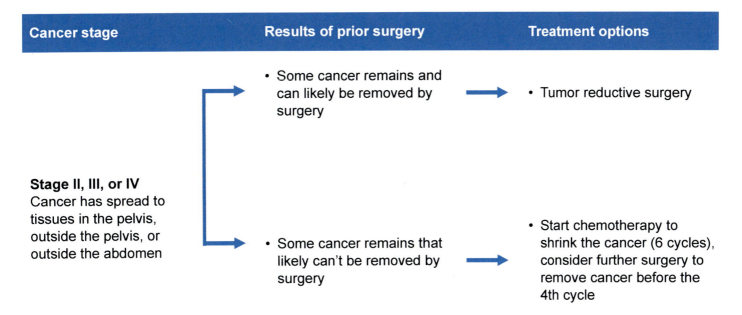

Cancer stage	Results of prior surgery	Treatment options
Stage II, III, or IV Cancer has spread to tissues in the pelvis, outside the pelvis, or outside the abdomen	• Some cancer remains and can likely be removed by surgery	• Tumor reductive surgery
	• Some cancer remains that likely can't be removed by surgery	• Start chemotherapy to shrink the cancer (6 cycles), consider further surgery to remove cancer before the 4th cycle

NCCN Guidelines for Patients®:
Ovarian Cancer, Version 1.2017

5 Treatment guide — Stages II, III, and IV ovarian cancer

Guide 8. Treatment after surgery for stages II, III, and IV ovarian cancer

Cancer stage	Adjuvant treatment options
Stage II or III Cancer has spread to nearby organs and tissues in the pelvis, or it has spread to tissues in the abdomen **Stage IV** Cancer has spread outside the abdomen to organs and tissues in other parts of the body	• Chemotherapy given in the abdomen (IP), or • Chemotherapy given in a vein (IV) for a total of 6 cycles • Completion surgery based on tumor response and possibility or being able to remove the cancer (certain patients)

Chemotherapy regimens for stage II, III, and IV ovarian cancer

Chemotherapy regimens	Route given	Length of a cycle
Paclitaxel and cisplatin	Injection in a vein (IV) and abdomen (IP)	21 days (3 weeks)
Paclitaxel and carboplatin	Injection in a vein (IV) and abdomen (IP)	21 days (3 weeks)
Dose-dense paclitaxel and carboplatin	Injection in a vein (IV)	21 days (3 weeks)
Paclitaxel and carboplatin	Injection in a vein (IV)	7 days (1 week)
Docetaxel and carboplatin	Injection in a vein (IV)	21 days (3 weeks)
Carboplatin and liposomal doxorubicin	Injection in vein (IV)	28 days (4 weeks)
Bevacizumab with paclitaxel and carboplatin	Injection in a vein (IV)	21 days (3 weeks)

Guide 8 shows the options that are recommended after surgery for stage II, III, or IV ovarian cancer. Most women with ovarian cancer will receive chemotherapy after primary treatment with surgery. This is called adjuvant treatment. Your doctor may also refer to this as primary chemotherapy.

There are a few adjuvant treatment options to choose from. Which option is best for you depends on the cancer stage and how much cancer is left after surgery. The cancer stage is a rating of how much the cancer has grown and spread. The goal of surgery is to not leave behind any tumors that are 1 cm or larger.

5 Treatment guide | Stages II, III, and IV ovarian cancer

Treatment options

For stage II or III ovarian cancer, the treatment options depend on how much cancer is left after surgery. If no tumors 1 cm or larger remain, then you have two options to choose from. One option is to receive chemotherapy given in the abdomen and some in the vein. The second option is to receive all your chemotherapy given in a vein. If any remaining tumors are 1 cm or larger, then you will receive chemotherapy given in a vein. For stage IV ovarian cancer, you will receive chemotherapy given in a vein.

Chemotherapy given in the abdomen is called IP chemotherapy. Chemotherapy given in a vein is called IV chemotherapy. It is important to discuss the differences between IP and IV chemotherapy with your doctor.

Even if you had some chemotherapy before surgery, you will likely have more chemotherapy after surgery. A total of 6 to 8 chemotherapy cycles is recommended for stage II, III, and IV ovarian cancer. If you had 3 cycles before surgery, at least three more cycles of chemotherapy after surgery is recommended.

Guide 8 also lists the chemotherapy regimens that are recommended for stage II, III, and IV ovarian cancer. Which drug or regimen is best for you depends on a number of factors. This includes your age, overall health, and performance status—a rating of how well you are able to do daily activities. Another key factor is your risk for peripheral neuropathy—a nerve problem that causes pain, tingling, and numbness typically in the hands and feet.

Neuropathy is a common side effect of paclitaxel and to a less degree carboplatin. If you have a high risk for nerve problems, then docetaxel and carboplatin may be a better option for you.

Some patients may not be able to tolerate the severe side effects of chemotherapy. This includes patients who are older than 65, have other health problems, or have trouble doing daily activities. For these patients, paclitaxel and carboplatin given once a week may be a good option. Giving these drugs once a week may cause fewer side effects than when they are given once every three weeks. It may be better tolerated by certain patients.

It is important that your kidneys are working well if you may receive a combination of IV and IP chemotherapy. Your doctor may give a blood test to check for chemicals that your kidneys filter out of your blood. High levels of certain chemicals may be a sign that your kidneys aren't working well. If you have trouble doing daily activities, have a high risk for neuropathy, or your kidneys aren't working well, then IP chemotherapy may not be a good treatment option for you.

Testing during chemotherapy treatment

During treatment, your doctor will give tests to see how well the chemotherapy is working and to check for side effects. A physical and pelvic exam should be done at least every 2 to 3 cycles. You may also have other tests as needed. This may include imaging tests, CBC, blood chemistry profile, and tests of CA-125 or other tumor markers.

Your doctor will also give some tests after chemotherapy treatment is finished to check how well it worked. An outcome or improvement related to treatment is called a treatment response. Once the treatment response is known, more treatment options may be considered.

5 Treatment guide — Stages II, III, and IV ovarian cancer

Guide 9. Treatment after primary chemotherapy

Chemotherapy results	Treatment options
Complete response — Tests show that the cancer is completely gone; all signs and symptoms have disappeared	• Clinical trial or • Observation with follow-up tests or • Maintenance treatment with pazopanib or • Maintenance treatment with paclitaxel
Partial response — The cancer has improved but it's not completely gone; some signs and symptoms remain	• Clinical trial and/or • Start recurrence treatment and/or • Best supportive care
Persistent or progressive disease — The cancer stayed the same or it continued to grow during treatment	• Clinical trial and/or • Best supportive care and/or • Start recurrence treatment

Guide 9 shows the options that are recommended after primary chemotherapy for stage II, III, or IV ovarian cancer. The next options depend on how well primary chemotherapy worked. An outcome or improvement related to treatment is called a treatment response.

A complete response is when there are no signs of cancer on the imaging tests, physical exam, or CA-125 blood tests after treatment. A partial response is when tests show a decrease in the amount of cancer, tumor size, or CA-125 levels. It means that the cancer improved, but it is not completely gone. Persistent disease is cancer that stayed the same—didn't get better or worse—during treatment. Progressive disease is cancer that continued to grow (progress) during or after treatment.

Treatment options

If tests showed a complete response, then you have four main options to choose from. The first option is to receive treatment within a clinical trial. A clinical trial is a type of research that studies how safe and helpful a treatment is. The second option is to begin observation with follow-up tests. Observation is a period of testing to watch for cancer growth after treatment. Another option is to begin maintenance treatment with paclitaxel or pazopanib. Maintenance treatment is given to continue (maintain) good treatment results.

For maintenance treatment, paclitaxel is given in a vein on Day 1 of a 28-day cycle for a total of 12 cycles. But, not all doctors recommend paclitaxel as maintenance treatment. It is important to discuss the benefits and risks with your doctor.

5 Treatment guide | Stages II, III, and IV ovarian cancer

If tests showed a partial response or persistent or progressive disease, then you have three main options to choose from. The first option is to receive treatment within a clinical trial. A second option is to start recurrence treatment—drugs given after prior treatments failed to kill all the cancer or keep it away.

Another option is to receive best supportive care. Supportive care is treatment given to relieve the symptoms of cancer or side effects of cancer treatment. It aims to improve quality of life and relieve any discomfort you have. Supportive care may be given alone. It may also be given along with recurrence treatment or treatment within a clinical trial.

5 Treatment guide | Follow-up after initial treatment

Follow-up after initial treatment

Guide 10. Follow-up testing after treatment

Follow-up tests and schedule

Follow-up visits every 2 to 4 months for 2 years, then every 3 to 6 months for 3 years, then once a year after 5 years with:

- Physical exam and pelvic exam

- CA-125 blood test or other tumor markers if initial results were high

- CBC and blood chemistry profile as needed

- CT, MRI, PET/CT of the chest, abdomen, and pelvis, or PET (bottom of the skull to mid-thigh) as needed

- Chest x-ray as needed

- Long-term wellness care

Guide 10 shows the follow-up tests that are recommended during observation and after completing cancer treatment. Observation is a period of testing to watch for cancer growth. Follow-up tests are used to check for signs of cancer return (relapse) or spread (metastasis). Doctors also use follow-up tests to monitor your health and check for side effects of treatment.

Follow-up tests

Follow-up tests are recommended every 2 to 4 months for 2 years, then every 3 to 6 months for 3 years, then once a year. Many of the tests used for follow-up will be the same as those used to find and confirm (diagnose) ovarian cancer.

The physical exam and pelvic exam help your doctor check for physical signs that the cancer has come back. Such signs may include swelling or bloating in your belly, abnormal lumps, or sudden changes in weight.

Blood tests to measure CA-125 or other tumor markers are recommended if levels were high when the cancer was first found. Rising CA-125 levels after treatment may be an early sign that the cancer has come back.

A CBC measures the number of each type of blood cell in a sample of blood. A blood chemistry profile may be done to check the health of certain organs and body systems.

Imaging tests of your chest, abdomen, and pelvis may be used to check if the cancer has spread. A CT, MRI, PET, or PET/CT scan may be used. A chest x-ray may be used to show if cancer has spread to your lungs. If you had fertility-sparing surgery, then ultrasound may be used to check for cancer in the other ovary. Once you are finished having babies, you should have surgery to remove the remaining ovary, fallopian tube, and uterus. This is called completion surgery.

5 Treatment guide | Follow-up after initial treatment

Guide 11. Treatment for ovarian cancer that has come back

Follow-up results	Prior treatment	Treatment options
Symptoms, imaging tests, or rising CA-125 levels signal that cancer has come back	• No prior chemotherapy	• Surgical treatment with or without chemotherapy
Clinical and/or radiographic relapse (symptoms and/or imaging test results show signs that cancer has come back after a complete response)	• Currently on chemotherapy (disease keeps growing)	• Clinical trial and/or • Best supportive care and/or • Start recurrence treatment
	• Finished chemotherapy <6 months ago	• Clinical trial and/or • Start recurrence treatment and/or • Best supportive care
	• Finished chemotherapy ≥6 months ago	Clinical and/or radiographic relapse: Maybe more surgery, then • Clinical trial and/or • Platinum-based chemotherapy for 6 cycles (preferred) or • Other recurrence treatment and/or • Best supportive care
Biochemical relapse (increase in CA-125 levels is the only sign that cancer has come back)	• Prior chemotherapy	• Clinical trial or • Delay recurrence treatment until symptoms appear (clinical relapse) or • Start recurrence treatment now, this may include platinum-based chemotherapy or • Best supportive care

5 Treatment guide | Follow-up after initial treatment

Genetic counseling is also recommended if it was not done before treatment. Genetic counseling is a discussion with a health expert about the risk for a disease caused by changes in genes. This is recommended because some health problems, including ovarian cancer, can run in families. New targeted therapies may also be available for woman with certain genetic mutations. Thus, it is important for you to know if you have any genetic mutations.

Guide 11 (on page 59) shows the options for ovarian cancer that has come back after prior treatment. The return of cancer after treatment is called a recurrence or relapse. The treatment options are based on the type of relapse and whether or not you've had chemotherapy before.

A biochemical relapse is when CA-125 levels are increased, but you don't have any symptoms and imaging tests show no signs that cancer has come back. A radiographic relapse is when imaging tests show signs that the cancer has come back. A clinical relapse is when you have symptoms that signal the cancer has come back. Symptoms of a relapse include pain or bloating in your pelvis or belly, unexplained weight loss, upset stomach, constipation, trouble eating or feeling full fast, fatigue, and needing to urinate often or urgently.

Once follow-up tests or symptoms signal a relapse, you may have imaging tests if they weren't done recently. This may include a CT, MRI, PET, or PET/CT scan of your chest, abdomen, and pelvis.

Treatment options

If cancer comes back and you haven't had chemotherapy yet, then the options are the same as those used for newly diagnosed ovarian cancer. This means that you will have surgery to remove the cancer and chemotherapy may be given next. The type and extent of surgery depends on how far the cancer has spread. If it looks like the cancer is only in your pelvis, then surgical staging may be done.

If it looks like the cancer has spread outside your pelvis, then you will have surgery to remove as much cancer as possible.

For a biochemical relapse after prior chemotherapy (elevated CA-125 tumor marker level but no other evidence of recurrence), there are some options to choose from. The preferred option is to join a clinical trial. A clinical trial is a type of research that studies how safe and helpful a test or treatment is.

For a clinical or radiographic relapse after chemotherapy, the options depend on long it's been since you finished treatment. If you finished chemotherapy less than 6 months ago, there are three options to choose from. The first option is to receive treatment within a clinical trial. The second option is to start recurrence treatment. The third option is to receive best supportive care. Supportive care is treatment given to relieve the symptoms of cancer or side effects of cancer treatment. It aims to improve quality of life and relieve any discomfort you have. Supportive care may be given alone. It may also be given along with recurrence treatment or treatment within a clinical trial.

If you finished chemotherapy at least 6 months ago, then you may have surgery to remove as much of the cancer as possible. After surgery, or without surgery, you still have other options to choose from. One option is to receive treatment within a clinical trial. The second option is to receive platinum-based chemotherapy as recurrence treatment. This is the preferred option especially for the first recurrence. The third option is to receive a different type of drug for recurrence treatment. Best supportive care is also recommended.

The second option is to wait and not start treatment until you have symptoms of a relapse. The third option is to start recurrence treatment right away, which may not be chemotherapy. Best supportive care is also recommended.

5 Treatment guide | Follow-up after initial treatment

Guide 12. Recurrence treatment

Preferred options

If cancer is platinum-sensitive:

- Carboplatin
- Carboplatin/docetaxel
- Carboplatin/gemcitabine
- Carboplatin/gemcitabine/bevacizumab
- Carboplatin/liposomal doxorubicin
- Carboplatin/paclitaxel, albumin bound (for patients with taxane hypersensitivity)
- Carboplatin/paclitaxel
- Carboplatin/paclitaxel (weekly)
- Cisplatin
- Cisplatin/gemcitabine

If cancer is platinum-resistant:

- Docetaxel
- Etoposide (oral)
- Gemcitabine
- Liposomal doxorubicin
- Liposomal doxorubicin/bevacizumab
- Paclitaxel (weekly) ± pazopanib
- Paclitaxel (weekly)/bevacizumab
- Topotecan
- Topotecan/bevacizumab

Targeted therapy (single agent)

- Bevacizumab
- Olaparib
- Rucaparib (if cancer is platinum-resistant)

Other options

- Altretamine
- Aromatase inhibitors
- Capecitabine
- Cyclophosphamide
- Carboplatin/paclitaxel/bevacizumab (if cancer is plantinum-sensitive)
- Doxorubicin
- Ifosfamide
- Irinotecan
- Leuprolide acetate
- Megestrol acetate

- Melphalan
- Oxaliplatin
- Palliative radiation therapy
- Paclitaxel
- Paclitaxel, albumin-bound
- Pazopanib
- Pemetrexed
- Rucaparib (if cancer is plantinum-sensitive)
- Tamoxifen
- Vinorelbine

5 Treatment guide | Follow-up after initial treatment

Guide 12 (on page 61) shows the options that are recommended for recurrence treatment. Recurrence treatment is given after prior chemotherapy treatment failed to kill all of the cancer or keep it away. Recurrence treatments include chemotherapy, hormone therapy, and targeted therapy drugs. (See Part 4 for more details about each type of drug.) Which option is best for you depends on a number of factors, including the type and length of the treatment response to prior chemotherapy.

Recurrence treatment is used to treat ovarian cancer that has come back after a partial or complete response to prior chemotherapy. It is also used to treat ovarian cancer that did not respond or continued to grow during prior chemotherapy treatment. When cancer comes back after a complete response, the options depend on how long it has been since chemotherapy ended.

Cancer is called "platinum-resistant" if the relapse happens less than 6 months after the last chemotherapy treatment. This means that platinum-based chemotherapy drugs such as cisplatin and carboplatin did not work very well against the cancer. Therefore a different type of drug is recommended for recurrence treatment.

Cancer is called "platinum-sensitive" if the relapse happens at least 6 or more months after the last chemotherapy treatment. This means that platinum-based chemotherapy drugs worked well against the cancer. Therefore, you may receive platinum-based chemotherapy again as recurrence treatment. This is the preferred option, especially if it is the first recurrence. But, other types of drugs may also be considered. See Guide 12.

In some cases, chemotherapy is combined with a targeted therapy like bevacizumab. Bevacizumab may be given with carboplatin and either gemcitabine or paclitaxel. If the bevacizumab continues after the chemotherapy is done, it is called maintenance therapy. Bevacizumab may continue until the disease or side effects worsen.

Maintenance therapy is given to continue (maintain) good results of prior treatment. Another example of maintenance therapy is a newly approved targeted agent called niraparib. This drug is considered for maintenance therapy after recurrence treatment. Niraparib may be an option for patients with platinum-sensitive disease that has a partial or complete response after recurrence treatment.

6 Treatment guide for LCOH (less common types of ovarian histopathologies)

64 Carcinosarcoma (MMMT [malignant mixed Müllerian tumor]

66 Clear cell carcinoma of the ovary

67 Mucinous carcinoma of the ovary

68 Low-grade (grade 1) serous/endometrioid epithelial carcinoma

70 Borderline epithelial tumors (LMP [low malignant potential]

74 Malignant sex cord-stromal tumors

76 Malignant germ cell tumors

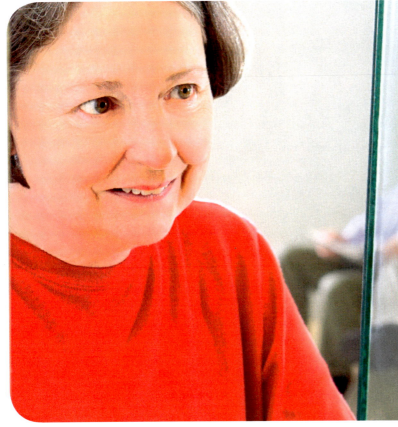
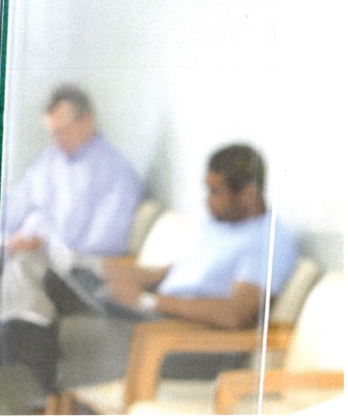

6 Treatment guide | Carcinosarcoma (MMMT)

Part 6 is a guide through the treatment options for people with less common types of ovarian cancer. It shows which tests and treatments are recommended under which conditions. This treatment information may help you ask your doctor questions about your next steps of care.

This information is taken from the treatment guidelines written by NCCN experts of ovarian cancer. These treatment guidelines list options for people with ovarian cancer in general. Thus, your doctors may suggest other treatment for you based on your health and personal needs. Discuss and decide on your treatment plan with your doctor.

Carcinosarcoma (MMMT [malignant mixed Müllerian tumor)

MMMTs are a rare type of ovarian tumor. Most doctors consider this less common ovarian cancer histopathology to be a type of poorly differentiated epithelial ovarian cancer. This means the cells may have changed form and become a MMMT.

When cancer is poorly differentiated, this means the cells look very different from normal cells when viewed under a microscope. Because the cells are "poorly" differentiated, the cancer may grow and spread more quickly. This type of cancer is considered aggressive. Thus, the first treatment option is surgery.

6 Treatment guide — Carcinosarcoma (MMMT)

Guide 13. Carcinosarcoma (MMMT [malignant mixed Müllerian tumor] of the ovary

Diagnosis	Stage	Adjuvant treatment options
Complete surgical staging	Stage I-IV	• Chemotherapy (same used for epithelial, preferred) or • Cisplatin + ifosfamide or • Carboplatin + ifosfamide or • Paclitaxel + ifosfamide

Guide 13 shows that surgery is the main treatment for a MMMT. Once surgery is complete and the cancer stage is known, other treatment may be offered. This next treatment is known as adjuvant treatment — treatment given after the primary (first) treatment for MMMT.

Adjuvant treatment options include different types of chemotherapy. Some patients may benefit from using the same types of chemotherapy drugs recommended for epithelial ovarian cancer. This may include the option of getting an IP regimen of cisplatin and paclitaxel. See Guide 8 on page 54 for a list of chemotherapy drugs that may be recommended. Other drug combinations given as adjuvant treatment include cisplatin and ifosfamide, carboplatin and ifosfamide, or paclitaxel and ifosfamide.

Surveillance and follow-up care follows the same path as for epithelial ovarian cancer. See Guides 10 and 11 for follow-up tests, test results, and next steps of care. Further treatment may be needed if the cancer comes back (recurs). Your doctor will follow you closely to watch for any signs or symptoms of disease. If more treatment is needed, options may include a clinical trial, recurrence treatment, and/or best supportive.

6 Treatment guide | Clear cell carcinoma of the ovary

Clear cell carcinoma of the ovary

Guide 14. Clear cell carcinoma of the ovary

Stage	Adjuvant treatment options
Stage IA-IC	• IV taxane/carboplatin for 3 to 6 cycles
Stage II-IV	• Chemotherapy (same used for epithelial)
Borderline	• See Guide 17 and 18

Clear cell is one of the subtypes of epithelial ovarian cancer. Most epithelial ovarian cancers are the serous subtype. The two other subtypes are mucinous (see Guide 15) and endometriod (see Guide 16). Clear cell is considered to be high grade. Thus, it may grow and spread more quickly.

Guide 14 shows the stage and adjuvant treatment options for clear cell carcinoma of the ovary. After completion surgery, surgical staging, and possible lymph node removal more treatment may follow. Lymph node removal has been shown to be beneficial for patients with this type of disease.

Adjuvant treatment options include chemotherapy for stage IA to IV clear cell carcinoma of the ovary. For stage IA to IC, an IV taxane (ie, docetaxel or paclitaxel) and carboplatin is given for 3 to 6 cycles. For stage II to IV, adjuvant treatment may have similar options like those given to treat epithelial ovarian cancer. (See Guide 8 on page 54 for possible treatment options).

If the disease is considered borderline, treatment options may include those recommended in Guides 17 and 18 for borderline epithelial tumors. The adjuvant treatment options are fertility-sparing surgery, observation, hormone therapy, or chemotherapy.

6 Treatment guide — Mucinous carcinoma of the ovary

Mucinous carcinoma of the ovary

Guide 15. Mucinous carcinoma of the ovary

Diagnosis	Stage	Adjuvant treatment options
If not done before: • GI tests • CEA (**c**arcino**e**mbryonic **a**ntigen) blood test • Consider surgical staging	• Stage IA-IB	• Observe or • If not done before, fertility-sparing surgery for certain patients
	• Stage IC	• Observe or • IV taxane/carboplatin for 3 to 6 cycles or • 5-FU + leucovorin + oxaliplatin or • Capecitabine + oxaliplatin or • If not done before, fertility-sparing surgery for certain patients
	• Stage II-IV	• Chemotherapy or • 5-FU + leucovorin + oxaliplatin or • Capecitabine + oxaliplatin
	• Borderline	• See Guides 17 and 18

Mucinous carcinoma of the ovary is usually diagnosed early on. This cancer involves large tumors that tend to fill the whole belly (abdomen) and pelvic area. The diagnosis occurs at a young age; usually at 20 to 40 years. Most people with mucinous carcinoma of the ovary respond well to treatment.

Mucinous carcinoma of the ovary is usually diagnosed after surgery for a suspicious tumor in the belly and pelvic area. The same tests that are ordered to diagnose other ovarian cancer are used for mucinous tumors. See Part 2, *Testing for ovarian cancer*.

6 Treatment guide | Low-grade serous/endometrioid epithelial

Guide 15 starts with more tests used to further diagnose mucinous carcinoma of the ovary. The GI tests and CEA blood test help doctors assess if the cancer started in the GI area and spread to the ovaries (metastatic cancer), or if the cancer started in the ovaries (primary cancer). Surgical staging is also done and gives more information about the extent of the cancer.

An appendectomy is also recommended during surgery for those with a mucinous carcinoma of the ovary. An appendectomy is the removal of the appendix. This organ is found at the beginning of the large intestine. It is located in the lower right side of your abdomen.

Once surgery is complete and the stage is known, adjuvant treatment may be offered. This includes observation, chemotherapy, and if not done before for stage IC, fertility-sparing surgery. Observation is an option for early-stage disease.

For stage IC, adjuvant treatment options are observation, IV carboplatin with either paclitaxel or docetaxel, 5-FU, leucovorin and oxaliplatin, or capecitabine/oxaliplatin. For stages II to IV adjuvant treatment may include chemotherapy (same given for epithelial ovarian cancer), 5-FU, leucovorin, and oxaliplatin, or capecitabine and oxaliplatin.

Some doctors think that the combinations of 5-FU, leucovorin, and oxaliplatin and capecitabine and oxaliplatin are helpful because these mucinous tumors are similar to GI tumors. Treatment for GI cancer includes those combinations of chemotherapy.

Low-grade (grade 1) serous/endometrioid epithelial carcinoma

Serous and endometrioid are less common subtypes of epithelial ovarian cancer. Low-grade serous epithelial cancer is a slow-growing (indolent) cancer found at a younger age than those with a high-grade serous epithelial ovarian cancer.

Endometrioid epithelial carcinoma may be related to endometriosis. Endometriosis is a medical condition where tissue inside the uterus grows out into other nearby tissue or organs like the ovaries and fallopian tubes. When examined, endometrioid tumors look similar to malignant sex cord-stromal tumors. (See page 74 for more information on malignant sex-cord stromal tumors.)

Primary treatment includes completion surgery with surgical staging followed by adjuvant treatment. Most people are diagnosed with low-grade serous/endometrioid epithelial carcinoma after surgery.

6 Treatment guide — Low-grade serous/endometrioid epithelial

Guide 16. Low-grade (grade 1) serous/endometrioid epithelial carcinoma

Stage	Adjuvant treatment options
Stage IA-IB	• Observe
Stage IC-II	• Observe or • IV taxane/carboplatin for 3 to 6 cycles or • Hormone therapy
Stage III-IV	• Chemotherapy or • Hormone therapy
Borderline	• See Guides 17 and 18

Guide 16 covers adjuvant treatment options for stage I to IV, and borderline disease. For stages I and II, observation may be option. Chemotherapy is a treatment option for stage IC to IV, but low-grade serous/endometrioid epithelial carcinoma may not respond as well to this treatment. Stage IC to II chemotherapy may include IV carboplatin with either paclitaxel or docetaxel. Another recommended treatment is hormone therapy, which includes anastrozole, letrozole, leuprolide, or tamoxifen. Stage III to IV treatment options include chemotherapy (same given for epithelial ovarian cancer) or hormone therapy.

For those with borderline low-grade serous/endometrioid epithelial carcinoma, fertility-sparing surgery is an option. Adjuvant treatment options for borderline disease are listed in Guides 17 and 18. The options include observation, chemotherapy, or hormone therapy.

6 Treatment guide | Borderline epithelial tumors

Borderline epithelial tumors (LMP [low malignant potential]

Guide 17. Borderline epithelial tumors (LMP) with surgical staging

Results	Adjuvant treatment options
No invasive implants	• Observe
Invasive implants	• Observe or • Consider treatment for grade 1 (low-grade) serous epithelial carcinoma (see Guide 16)

This type of cancer is slow growing and may not invade other tissue. An LMP tumor may be found by chance during surgery or tests for another health problem. Most often, it is diagnosed after surgery. Surgery is also used as primary treatment for this type of tumor.

There is more than one primary treatment option for an LMP tumor. Your doctor will consider more than one factor when deciding on treatment. First, surgical staging will be done to assess the extent of disease. Second, your doctor will check whether or not invasive implants were found. Tumor cells that spread and grow on the surface of nearby organs are called noninvasive implants. The tumor cells rarely grow into (invade) tissue—called invasive implants. Lastly, he or she will factor in whether or not you want to have babies after treatment. Fertility-sparing surgery is always an option for an LMP tumor.

Observation with follow-up tests is an option for all patients. See Guide 17.

If surgical staging was complete and no invasive implants were found, then this is the only option recommended. If invasive implants were found, a second option is to receive chemotherapy. If surgical staging was not complete, then another option is to have more surgery. This may include fertility-sparing surgery and surgical staging procedures.

For surgical staging, biopsy samples will be taken from the tumor and nearby tissues. The omentum and nearby lymph nodes may also be removed. If you don't want to have babies, then you may have completion surgery. Completion surgery removes the remaining ovary (or ovaries), fallopian tubes, uterus, omentum, and any tumor cells found on nearby tissue. In some cases, nearby lymph nodes may also be removed.

If invasive implants were found, then surgery may be followed by chemotherapy. If no invasive implants were found, then no other treatment is recommended after either surgery. Instead, you will begin observation with follow-up tests.

6 Treatment guide — Borderline epithelial tumors

Guide 18. Borderline epithelial tumors (LMP) with incomplete surgical staging

Staging	Disease status	Adjuvant treatment options
CT of the chest, abdomen, and pelvis with contrast	• Residual disease remaining after surgical staging	**Fertility desired, no invasive implants or unknown:** • Observe or • Fertility-sparing surgery and removal of residual disease **Fertility desired, invasive implants at prior surgery:** • Fertility-sparing surgery and removal of residual disease or • Observe or • Consider treatment for grade 1 (low-grade) serous epithelial carcinoma (see Guide 16) **Fertility not desired, no invasive implants or unknown:** • Observe or • Completion surgery and removal of residual disease **Fertility not desired, invasive implants at prior surgery:** • Completion surgery and removal of residual disease or • Observe or • Consider treatment for grade 1 (low-grade) serous epithelial carcinoma (see Guide 16)
	• No residual disease remaining after surgical staging	• Observe

NCCN Guidelines for Patients®:
Ovarian Cancer, Version 1.2017

6 Treatment guide — Borderline epithelial tumors

Guide 19. Follow-up testing after treatment for borderline epithelial tumors (LMP)

Follow-up tests and schedule

Follow-up visits every 3 to 6 months for 5 years, then once a year with:

- Physical exam and pelvic exam
- CA-125 blood test or other tumor markers as needed
- CBC and blood chemistry profile as needed
- CT, MRI, PET/CT of the chest, abdomen, and pelvis, or PET (bottom of the skull to mid-thigh) as needed
- Ultrasound as needed if you had fertility-sparing surgery
- Completion surgery, if you had fertility-sparing surgery and are finished having babies

Guide 18 shows adjuvant treatment options if surgical staging was not complete. One option is to have more surgery. Fertility-sparing surgery is an option for patients with residual disease that remains after surgical staging. If you don't want to have babies, then you may have completion surgery. Completion surgery removes the remaining ovary (or ovaries), fallopian tubes, uterus, omentum, and any tumor cells found on nearby tissue. In some cases, nearby lymph nodes may also be removed.

If invasive implants were found, chemotherapy is another option for those who want or don't want fertility-sparing surgery. If no invasive implants were found, no systemic treatment is recommended after either surgery. You may begin observation or have fertility-sparing surgery with removal of residual disease.

Guide 19 shows the follow-up tests that are recommended during observation and after primary treatment for an LMP tumor. Observation is a period of testing to watch for tumor growth. Follow-up tests are given on a regular basis to watch for signs that tumor cells have come back or spread after treatment. Many of the follow-up tests are the same as those used to find and confirm the tumor.

Follow-up visits are recommended every 3 to 6 months for 5 years. After that, they are recommended once a year. A physical exam and pelvic exam should be done at every follow-up visit. These exams help your doctor check for physical signs that the tumor has come back. Such signs may include swelling or bloating in your belly, abnormal lumps, or sudden changes in weight. Blood tests to measure CA-125 or other tumor markers are recommended if levels were high when the tumor was first found. Rising CA-125 levels after treatment may be an early sign that the tumor has come back. A CBC measures the number of each type of blood cell in a sample of blood. A blood chemistry profile may be done to check the health of certain organs and body systems.

Ultrasound uses sound waves to make pictures of the inside of the body. It may be used to look for signs of tumor growth if you had fertility-sparing surgery. This type of surgery only removes one ovary and its fallopian tube so that you will still be able to have babies. Once you are finished having babies, you should have completion surgery.

6 Treatment guide — Borderline epithelial tumors

Guide 20. Treatment for borderline epithelial tumors (LMP) tumor relapse

Follow-up results	Next steps	Treatment options
Clinical relapse Relapse based on symptoms, imaging test results, or increase in CA-125 levels	• Surgical evaluation and • Debulking if needed	**If no invasive implants** • Observe **If invasive implants or low-grade invasive carcinoma** • See Guide 16 for grade 1 (low-grade) serous epithelial carcinoma options **Invasive carcinoma (high-grade)** • See Part 5 for treatment of epithelial ovarian cancer

Guide 20 shows the treatment options for an LMP tumor that has come back after treatment. This is called a recurrence or relapse. After a clinical relapse, you may have surgery so that your doctor can see where the tumor has spread. This is called surgical evaluation. You may also have surgery to remove as much of the tumor as possible. This is called debulking surgery.

The treatment options for a relapse depend on whether or not tumor cells have grown into (invaded) nearby tissues. These are called invasive implants. If there aren't any invasive implants, then observation with follow-up tests is recommended. If there are invasive implants or invasive (high-grade) carcinoma, then you have two treatment options to choose from. One option is to have surgery followed by chemotherapy, as described for primary treatment in Part 5, *Treatment guide for epithelial ovarian cancer*.

6 Treatment guide — Malignant sex cord-stromal tumors

Malignant sex cord-stromal tumors

Guide 21. Malignant sex cord-stromal tumors

Staging	Adjuvant treatment options
Stage IA to IC • Fertility sparing surgery with complete staging → Stage I low risk	• Observe
→ Stage I high risk or • Intermediate risk	• Observe or • Consider platinum-based chemotherapy
All others • Complete staging → Stage II-IV	• Platinum-based chemotherapy or • Radiation for limited disease

Malignant sex cord-stromal tumors include granulosa cell tumors and Sertoli-Leydig cell tumors. Granulosa cell tumors are the more common of the two. Malignant sex cord-stromal tumors are rare. Malignant sex cord-stromal tumors are usually a slow-growing (indolent) type of ovarian cancer. It is often found at an early stage of disease.

Guide 21 starts with staging of sex cord-stromal tumors. If you want to have babies after treatment, fertility-sparing surgery is offered with complete staging. Once the stage is known, patients with stage I disease are referred to as low risk or high risk. Those with low risk may be observed. Those with stage I high risk or intermediate (middle) risk may be observed or get a platinum-based chemotherapy. For stage II to IV, platinum-based chemotherapy or radiation to a limited area is recommended.

Chemotherapy drugs given to treat malignant sex cord-stromal tumors include BEP (**b**leomycin, **e**toposide, and **c**isplatin), as well as paclitaxel and cisplatin or carboplatin. If you are prescribed bleomycin, pulmonary function tests may be before treatment. The pulmonary function tests will check to see if your lungs are working properly.

6 Treatment guide | Malignant sex cord-stromal tumors

Guide 22. Treatment for malignant sex cord-stromal tumor relapse

Follow-up results	Recurrence treatment options
Clinical relapse of stage II-IV Relapse based on symptoms, imaging test results, or increase in CA-125 levels	• Clinical trial or • Consider secondary cytoreductive surgery or • Recurrence treatment

Guide 22 shows the treatment options for a sex cord-stromal tumor that has come back after treatment. This is called a recurrence or relapse. Symptoms, imaging tests, and a CA-125 blood test will confirm a clinical relapse. After a clinical relapse, you have the option to join a clinical trial, consider more surgery (cytoreductive), or get recurrence treatment. Cytoreductive surgery may remove all or part of organs or tissues the cancer has spread to. This is also called debulking surgery.

6 Treatment guide — Malignant germ cell tumors

Malignant germ cell tumors

Guide 23. Malignant germ cell tumors with surgical staging

Diagnosis	Treatment options
Initial surgery • Fertility desired	• Fertility-sparing surgery and comprehensive staging
Initial surgery • Fertility not desired	• Completion staging surgery
Prior surgery • Completely staged	• See Guides 25 and 26 for treatment options per stage

Malignant germ cell tumors include malignant tumors, dysgerminomas, immature teratomas, embryonal tumors, and endodermal sinus (yolk sac) tumors. These tumors are usually diagnosed between the ages of 16 and 20 years. They are often stage I at diagnosis. Germ cell tumors respond well to treatment.

Initial testing for germ cell tumors may include pulmonary function tests to check your breathing. This is done before giving a drug like bleomycin. Your AFP (**a**lpha-**f**eto**p**rotein) level is also checked and can be found in the blood when germ cell tumors are present.

Guide 23 details surgery for germ cell tumors. Surgery is the primary treatment option for germ cell tumors. Surgical staging and fertility-sparing surgery are also options. If you don't want to have babies, then completion surgery is the type of surgery you will have.

6 Treatment guide | Malignant germ cell tumors

Guide 24. Malignant germ cell tumors with incomplete surgical staging

Diagnosis	Test results	Treatment options
Dysgerminoma or Grade 1 immature teratoma	• Positive imaging and positive tumor markers	**Fertility desired** • Fertility-sparing surgery and comprehensive staging **Fertility not desired** • Completion staging surgery
	• Negative imaging and positive tumor markers	• Consider observation
	• Negative imaging and negative tumor markers	• Consider observation
Embryonal, endodermal sinus tumor (yolk sac tumor), grade 2-3 immature teratoma, or mixed histology	• Positive imaging and positive tumor markers	**Fertility desired** • Fertility-sparing surgery and comprehensive staging **Fertility not desired** • Completion staging surgery with possible tumor reductive surgery or • Chemotherapy
	• Negative imaging and positive or negative tumor markers	• See Guide 25 for treatment options per stage

Guide 24 covers diagnosis, tests results, and treatment options for germ cell tumors. If diagnosed with dysgerminoma or grade 1 immature teratoma, you will have imaging tests and blood tests (tumor markers will be measured). Tumor markers can be high in blood levels and indicate that cancer or another medical condition is present. Tumor markers cannot be used alone to diagnose cancer.

Your imaging and tumor marker test results will determine which treatment options you are offered. If positive on imaging and tumor marker tests, you will be offered fertility-sparing surgery and will have surgical staging. If you don't want to have babies, completion surgery will come next.

If you are negative on imaging and tumor marker tests, you will be observed.

For embryonal, endodermal sinus (yolk sac tumor), grade 2 to 3 immature teratoma, and tumors of mixed histology you will also have imaging and blood tests (tumor markers will be measured). If positive on imaging and tumor marker tests, you will be ~~are~~ offered fertility-sparing surgery and will have surgical staging. If you don't want to have babies, you will have completion surgery. If other remaining cancer can likely be removed, then tumor reductive surgery is recommended. Your doctor will remove as much of the cancer as possible This is called tumor reduction surgery.

NCCN Guidelines for Patients®:
Ovarian Cancer, Version 1.2017

6 Treatment guide — Malignant germ cell tumors

Guide 25. Malignant germ cell tumors adjuvant treatment options by stage

Stage	Adjuvant treatment options
Stage I dysgerminoa or Stage I, grade 1 immature teratoma	• Observe
Any stage embryonal tumor or Any stage endodermal sinus tumor (yolk sac tumor) or Stage II-IV dysgerminoma or Stage I, grade 2-3 or stage II-IV immature tertoma	• Chemotherapy

Guide 25 lists adjuvant treatment options for germ cell tumors. Observation is an option for stage 1 dysgerminoma and grade 1 immature teratoma. For embryonal, endodermal sinus (yolk sac tumor), stage II to IV dysgerminoma, and stage I grade 2 to 3 or stage II to IV immature teratoma, chemotherapy is recommended.

Chemotherapy drugs given for malignant germ cell tumors are bleomycin, etoposide, cisplatin, and carboplatin. These drugs are given as a combination treatment. Etoposide may be given with cisplatin or carboplatin.

6 Treatment guide — Malignant germ cell tumors

Guide 26. Possible response to chemotherapy for malignant germ cell tumors

Disease status	Follow-up care	Treatment options
Complete clinical response	Observe • If abnormal markers with definitive recurrent disease	• Consider chemotherapy or • High-dose chemotherapy
Residual tumor on imaging with normal tumor markers	Consider surgery or observe • If necrotic tissue	• Observe
	Consider surgery or observe • If benign teratoma	• CT of the chest, abdomen, and pelvis or MRI as needed
	Consider surgery or observe • If residual malignancy	• Consider more platinum-based chemotherapy for 2 cycles
Elevated tumor markers (persistent) with definitive residual disease		• TIP (paclitaxel + ifosfamide + cisplatin) or • High-dose chemotherapy (strong recommendation for care at a major hospital for possible stem-cell transplant and curative therapy)

Guide 26 shares the response to chemotherapy for germ cell tumors. A complete response is followed by observation and possible chemotherapy if disease comes back (recurs). If residual tumor remains and tumor markers are normal, surgery or observation is considered. If more information is needed after a benign (no cancer) teratoma is found, tests can be ordered, and you may be observed. If necrotic (dead) tissue is found, you may also be observed.

6 Treatment guide — Malignant germ cell tumors

Guide 27. Follow-up testing after treatment for malignant sex cord-stromal tumors and malignant germ cell tumors

Follow-up tests

- Physical exam

- CA-125 blood test or other tumor markers (after 2 years for malignant germ cell tumors, only as needed)

- Chest x-ray; CT of the chest, abdomen, and pelvis; MRI; PET/CT; or PET as needed for germ cell tumors only

- For concern of recurrence of malignant sex cord-stromal tumors and malignant germ cell tumors:
    - CT of the chest, abdomen, and pelvis with contrast. Other imaging tests can be considered like chest x-ray, MRI, PET/CT, or PET.
    - CA-125 blood test or other tumor markers

Guide 27 covers follow-up tests that are recommended every 2 to 4 months for 2 years for women with malignant sex cord-stromal tumors and malignant germ cell tumors. Those with malignant sex cord-stromal tumors then will have a physical exam and serum tumor marker test done every 6 months after 2 years. These tests may continue past 5 years if your doctor thinks they are necessary. A follow-up physical exam is done once a year, after 2 years treatment for malignant germ cell tumors.

The physical exam and pelvic exam help your doctor check for physical signs that the cancer has come back. Such signs may include swelling or bloating in your belly, abnormal lumps, or sudden changes in weight. Blood tests to measure CA-125 or other tumor markers are recommended to check for early signs that the cancer has come back.

Imaging tests of your chest, abdomen, and pelvis may be used to check if the cancer is present. An x-ray, CT, MRI, PET, or PET/CT scan may be used for germ cell tumors only. There are not enough scientific data for doctors to recommend regular imaging tests for malignant sex cord-stromal tumors.

If there is concern that the cancer has come back (recurred) for both malignant sex cord-stromal tumors and malignant germ cell tumors, a CT of the chest, abdomen, and pelvis with contrast may be considered. Other imaging tests can be also be done and include a chest x-ray, MRI, PET/CT, or PET. Your CA-125 level and other tumor markers may also be measured at this time.

7 Making treatment decisions

- 82 It's your choice
- 82 Questions to ask your doctors
- 86 Deciding between options
- 87 Websites
- 87 Review

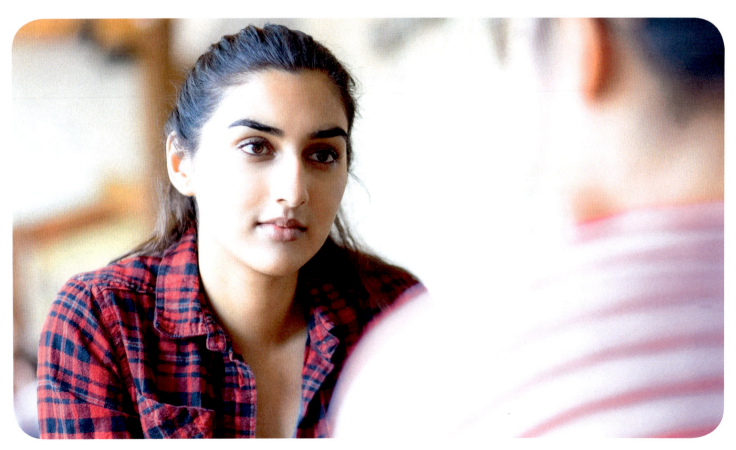

1 Making treatment decisions

It's your choice | Questions to ask

Finding out you have cancer can be very stressful. While absorbing the fact that you have cancer, you also must learn about tests and treatments. In addition, the time you have to decide on a treatment plan may feel short. Parts 1 through 6 aimed to teach you about ovarian cancer. Part 7 addresses ways to assist you when deciding on a treatment plan.

It's your choice

The role patients want in choosing their treatment differs. You may feel uneasy about making treatment decisions. This may be due to a high level of stress. It may be hard to hear or know what others are saying. Stress, pain, and drugs can limit your ability to make good decisions. You may feel uneasy because you don't know much about cancer. You've never heard the words used to describe cancer, tests, or treatments. Likewise, you may think that your judgment isn't any better than your doctors'.

Letting others decide which option is best may make you feel more at ease. However, whom do you want to make the decisions? You may rely on your doctors alone to make the right decisions. However, your doctors may not tell you which to choose if you have multiple good options. You can also have loved ones help. They can gather information, speak on your behalf, and share in decision-making with your doctors. Even if others decide which treatment you will receive, you still have to agree by signing a consent form.

On the other hand, you may want to take the lead or share in decision-making. In shared decision-making, you and your doctors share information, discuss the options, and agree on a treatment plan.

Your doctors know the science behind your plan but you know your concerns and goals. By working together, you can decide on a plan that works best for you when it comes to your personal and health needs.

Questions to ask your doctors

You will likely meet with experts from different fields of medicine. It is helpful to talk with each person. Prepare questions before your visit and ask questions if the information isn't clear. You can also get copies of your medical records. It may be helpful to have a family member or friend with you at these visits to listen carefully and even take notes. A patient advocate or navigator might also be able to come. They can help you ask questions and remember what was said.

The questions below are suggestions for information you read about in this book. Feel free to use these questions or come up with your own personal questions to ask your doctor and other members of your treatment team.

7 Making treatment decisions | Questions to ask your doctors

Questions to ask your doctors about testing

1. What tests will I have?

2. Where will the tests take place? Will I have to go to the hospital?

3. How long will it take? Will I be awake?

4. Will any test hurt?

5. What are the risks?

6. How do I prepare for testing?

7. Should I bring a list of my medications?

8. Should I bring someone with me?

9. How soon will I know the test results?

10. Who will explain the test results to me?

11. Can I have a copy of the test results and pathology report?

12. Who will talk with me about the next steps? When?

7 Making treatment decisions | Questions to ask your doctors

Questions to ask your doctors about treatment

1. What treatments do you recommend?

2. Will I have more than one treatment?

3. What are the risks and benefits of each treatment? What about side effects?

4. Will my age, general health, and other factors affect my treatment choices?

5. Would you help me get a 2nd opinion?

6. How soon should I start treatment? How long does treatment take?

7. Where will I be treated? Will I have to stay in the hospital or can I go home after each treatment?

8. What can I do to prepare for treatment?

9. What symptoms should I look out for during treatment?

10. How much will the treatment cost? How can I find out how much my insurance company will cover?

11. How likely is it that I'll be cancer-free after treatment?

12. What is the chance that the cancer will come back?

13. What should I do after I finish treatment?

14. Are there supportive services that I can get involved in? Support groups?

7 Making treatment decisions | Questions to ask your doctors

Questions to ask your doctors about clinical trials

1. What clinical trial is right for me?

2. What is the purpose of the study?

3. How many people will be in the clinical trial?

4. What are the tests and treatments for this study? And how often will they be?

5. Has the treatment been used before? Has it been used for other types of cancers?

6. What side effects can I expect from the treatment? Can the side effects be controlled?

7. How long will I be in the clinical trial?

8. Will I be able to get other treatment if this treatment doesn't work?

9. How will you know the treatment is working?

10. Who will help me understand the costs of the clinical trial?

7 Making treatment decisions | Deciding between options

Deciding between options

Deciding which option is best can be hard. Doctors from different fields of medicine may have different opinions about which option is best for you. This can be very confusing. Your spouse or partner may disagree with which option you want. This can be stressful. In some cases, one option hasn't been shown to work better than another, so science isn't helpful. Some ways to decide on treatment are discussed next.

Getting a 2nd opinion

Even if you like and trust your doctor, it may be helpful to get a 2nd opinion. You will want to have another doctor review your test results. He or she can suggest a treatment plan or check the one you already heard about.

Things you can do to prepare:

- Check with your insurance company about its rules on 2nd opinions. You want to know about out-of-pocket costs for doctors who are not part of your insurance plan.

- Make plans to have copies of all your records sent to the doctor you will see for your 2nd opinion. Do this well before your appointment. If you run into trouble having records sent, pick them up and bring them with you.

- If the new doctor offers other advice, make an appointment with your first doctor to talk about the differences. Do whatever you need to feel confident about your diagnosis and treatment plan.

Getting support

Support groups often include people at different stages of treatment. Some may be in the process of deciding while others may be finished with treatment. At support groups, you can ask questions and hear about the experiences of other people with ovarian cancer. If your hospital or community doesn't have support groups for people with ovarian cancer, check out the websites on the next page.

You can also reach out to a social worker or psychologist. They can help you find ways to cope or refer you to support services. These services may also be available to your family, friends, and those with children so they can connect and get support.

What to remember...

✓ Every treatment option has benefits and risks. Consider these when deciding which option is best for you.

✓ Talking to others may help identify benefits and risks you haven't thought of.

7 Making treatment decisions | Websites | Review

Websites

American Cancer Society
cancer.org/cancer/ovariancancer/index

Foundation for Women's Cancer
foundationforwomenscancer.org

National Cancer Institute
cancer.gov/types/ovarian/patient/ovarian-epithelial-treatment-pdq#section/_104

National Coalition for Cancer Survivorship
canceradvocacy.org/toolbox

National Ovarian Cancer Coalition
ovarian.org

NCCN
nccn.org/patients

Ovarian Cancer Research Fund Alliance
ocrfa.org

Sharsheret
sharsheret.org

The Society of Gynecologic Oncology
sgo.org

Review

> Shared decision-making is a process in which you and your doctors plan treatment together.

> Asking your doctors questions is vital to getting the information you need to make informed decisions.

> Getting a 2nd opinion, attending support groups, and comparing benefits and risks may help you decide which treatment is best for you.

My wife, Cathy, was diagnosed with Stage 3-C ovarian cancer in August 2011. Looking back, she recognized that she suffered symptoms for over a year before being diagnosed. During her battle with ovarian cancer, she fought to create earlier awareness initiatives. Although she is no longer with us, we will continue to make earlier awareness our foundation's focus.

*- Joel Van Antwerp
Catharine F. and Joel C. Van Antwerp Charitable Fund*

Glossary

89 Dictionary

95 Acronyms

Dictionary

abdomen
The belly area between the chest and pelvis.

adjuvant treatment
Treatment given after the main treatment used to rid the body of disease.

allergic reaction
Symptoms caused when the body is trying to rid itself of invaders.

ascites
Abnormal fluid buildup in the belly (abdomen) or pelvis.

bilateral salpingo-oophorectomy (BSO)
Surgery to remove both ovaries and both fallopian tubes.

biochemical relapse
A rise in CA-125 levels signals that cancer has come back after treatment.

biopsy
Removal of small amounts of tissue from the body to be tested for disease.

bladder
An organ that holds and expels urine from the body.

blood chemistry profile
A test that measures the amounts of many different chemicals in a sample of blood.

blood vessel
A tube that carries blood throughout the body.

borderline epithelial tumor (low malignant potential [LMP])
A tumor formed by abnormal cells that start in the epithelial cells of the ovary. This tumor type is slow growing and does not invade other tissue.

***BRCA1* or *BRCA2* genes**
Coded information in cells that help to prevent tumor growth by fixing damaged cells and helping cells grow normally. Abnormal changes within these genes increases the chances of developing breast and ovarian cancer.

cancer antigen 125 (CA-125)
A protein with sugar molecules on it that is made by ovarian cancer cells and normal cells.

cancer grade
A rating of how much the cancer cells look like normal cells.

cancer stage
A rating of the growth and spread of cancer in the body.

cancer staging
The process of rating and describing the extent of cancer in the body.

capsule
A thin layer of tissue that surrounds an organ—like the skin of an apple.

cell subtype
Smaller groups that at type of cancer is divided into based on how the cancer cells look under a microscope.

cervix
The lower part of the uterus that connects to the vagina.

chemotherapy
Drugs that kill fast-growing cells throughout the body, including normal cells and cancer cells.

chest x-ray
A test that uses x-rays to make pictures of the inside of the chest.

clear cell
One of the four main cell subtypes of ovarian cancer.

clinical relapse
Physical signs or symptoms signal that cancer has come back after treatment.

clinical trial
Research on a test or treatment to assess its safety or how well it works.

combination regimen
The use of two or more drugs.

complete blood count (CBC)
A test of the number of blood cells.

Dictionary

complete response
All signs and symptoms of cancer are gone after treatment.

completion surgery
Surgery to remove the remaining ovary, fallopian tube, uterus, and all cancer that can be seen.

computed tomography (CT) scan
A test that uses x-rays from many angles to make a picture of the inside of the body.

contrast
A dye put into your body to make clearer pictures during imaging tests.

cycle
Days of treatment followed by days of rest.

cytoreductive surgery
Surgery to remove as much cancer as possible. Also called debulking surgery.

debulking surgery
Surgery to remove as much cancer as possible. Also called cytoreductive surgery.

deoxyribonucleic acid (DNA)
Molecules that contain coded instructions for making and controlling cells.

diagnose
To identify a disease.

diagnosis
The process of identifying or confirming a disease.

diaphragm
The muscles below the ribs that help a person to breathe.

epithelial cells
Cells that form the outer layer of tissue around organs in the body.

epithelial ovarian cancer
Cancer that starts in the cells that form the outer layer of tissue around the ovaries.

fallopian tube
A thin tube through which an egg travels from the ovary to the uterus.

fatigue
Severe tiredness despite getting enough sleep.

fertility-sparing surgery
Surgery that only removes one ovary and fallopian tube so that a woman can still have babies.

follow-up test
Tests done after the start of treatment to check how well treatment is working.

gastrointestinal (GI) evaluation
A test to view the organs that food passes through when you eat.

gastrointestinal tract
The group of organs that food passes through when you eat.

general anesthesia
A controlled loss of wakefulness from drugs.

genes
A set of coded instructions in cells for making new cells and controlling how cells behave.

genetic counseling
A discussion with a health expert about the risk for a disease caused by changes in genes.

genetic counselor
A health expert that has special training to help patients understand changes in genes that are related to disease.

genetic testing
Tests to look for changes in coded instructions (genes) that increase the risk for a disease.

germ cell
Reproductive cells that become eggs in women and sperm in men.

gynecologic oncologist
A surgeon who's an expert in cancers that start in a woman's reproductive organs.

hereditary ovarian cancer
Ovarian cancer caused by abnormal coded information in cells that is passed down from parent to child.

hormone
Chemicals in the body that activate cells or organs.

Dictionary

hormone therapy
Treatment that stops the making or action of hormones in the body.

hot flashes
A health condition of intense body heat and sweat for short periods.

hysterectomy
Surgery to remove the uterus.

imaging test
Tests that make pictures (images) of the inside of the body.

implant
Cancer cells that broke away from the first tumor and formed new tumors on the surface of nearby organs and tissues.

infusion
A method of giving drugs slowly through a needle into a vein.

intestine
The organ that eaten food passes through after leaving the stomach.

intraperitoneal (IP) chemotherapy
Chemotherapy drugs given directly into the belly (abdomen) through a small tube.

intraperitoneal (IP)
Given directly into the belly (abdomen) through a small tube.

intravenous (IV) chemotherapy
Chemotherapy drugs given through a needle or tube inserted into a vein.

intravenous (IV)
Given by a needle or tube inserted into a vein.

invasion
When one kind of cell grows into organs or tissues where it doesn't belong.

invasive implant
Cancer cells that broke away from the first tumor and are growing into (invading) supporting tissue of nearby organs.

kidneys
A pair of organs that filter blood and remove waste from the body through urine.

laparotomy
Surgery with a long, up-and-down cut through the wall of the belly (abdomen).

large intestine
The organ that prepares unused food for leaving the body.

liver
An organ that removes waste from blood and makes a liquid that helps to digest food.

liver function test
A blood test that measures chemicals that are made or processed by the liver to check how well the liver is working.

lymph
A clear fluid containing white blood cells that fight infection and disease.

lymph nodes
Small groups of special disease-fighting cells located throughout the body.

lymph vessels
Small tubes that carry lymph—a clear fluid with white blood cells that fight infection and disease—throughout the body.

Lynch syndrome
Abnormal changes within genes that increase the chances of developing Colon, rectum, endometrial, ovarian, and other cancers. It is also called heredity non-polyposis colorectal cancer syndrome (HNPCC).

magnetic resonance imaging (MRI) scan
A test that uses radio waves and powerful magnets to make pictures of the inside of the body.

maintenance treatment
Treatment given to continue (maintain) good results of prior treatment.

medical history
All health events and medications taken to date.

medical oncologist
A doctor who is an expert in treating cancer with drugs such as chemotherapy.

menopause
The point in time when menstrual periods end.

menstrual cycle
Changes in the womb and ovaries that prepare a woman's body for pregnancy.

Dictionary

metastases
Tumors formed by cancer cells that have spread from the first tumor to other parts of the body.

metastasis
The spread of cancer cells from the first tumor to another body part.

microscope
A tool that uses lenses to see very small things the eyes can't.

microscopic metastases
Cancer cells that have spread from the first tumor to another body part and are too small to be seen with the naked eye.

mutation
An abnormal change in the instructions in cells for making and controlling cells.

neuropathy
A nerve problem that causes pain, tingling, and numbness in the hands and feet.

noninvasive implant
Cancer cells that broke away from the first tumor and are growing on the surface of nearby organs, but are not growing into (invading) tissue.

observation
A period of testing to watch for cancer growth.

omentum
The layer of fatty tissue that covers organs in the belly (abdomen).

ovaries
The pair of organs in women that make eggs for reproduction (making babies) and make hormones.

ovary
One of a pair of organs in women that make eggs for reproduction (making babies) and make hormones.

partial response
Cancer improved as a result of treatment—tests show a decrease in the amount of cancer, tumor size, or CA-125 levels—but it's not completely gone.

pathologist
A doctor who's an expert in testing cells and tissue to find disease.

pelvic exam
A medical exam of the female organs in the pelvis.

pelvis
The body area between the hip bones.

peritoneal cavity
The space inside the belly (abdomen) that contains abdominal organs such as the intestines, stomach, and liver.

peritoneal washing
A test in which a special liquid is used to wash the inside of the belly (peritoneal cavity) to check for cancer cells.

peritoneal washings
Sample of liquid that is tested for cancer cells after it is used to "wash" the inside of the belly (peritoneal cavity).

peritoneum
The layer of tissue that lines the inside of the belly (abdomen) and pelvis and covers most organs in this space.

persistent disease
Cancer that stayed the same—didn't get better or worse—during treatment.

physical exam
A review of the body by a health expert for signs of disease.

platinum agent
A cancer drug that is made with platinum. These drugs damage DNA in cells, which stops them from making new cells and causes them to die.

platinum-based chemotherapy
Treatment with two or more chemotherapy drugs and the main drug is made with platinum. Such drugs include cisplatin and carboplatin.

platinum-resistant
When cancer drugs made with platinum, such as cisplatin and carboplatin, do not work well against the cancer.

platinum-sensitive
When cancer drugs made with platinum, such as cisplatin and carboplatin, work well against the cancer.

poly ADP-ribose polymerase (PARP)
A protein that helps repair damaged DNA in cells.

positron emission tomography (PET) scan
A test that uses a sugar radiotracer—a form of sugar that is put into your body and lets off a small amount of energy that is absorbed by active cells—to view the shape and function of organs and tissues inside your body.

Dictionary

positron emission tomography (PET)/computed tomography (CT) scan
A test that uses a sugar radiotracer and x-rays from many angles to view the shape and function of organs and tissues inside the body.

primary chemotherapy
The first or main chemotherapy drugs given to treat cancer.

primary treatment
The main treatment used to rid the body of cancer.

primary tumor
The first mass of cancer cells in the body.

prognosis
The likely or expected course and outcome of a disease.

progressive disease
Cancer that continued to grow (progress) during or after treatment.

radiographic relapse
Imaging tests show signs that cancer has come back after treatment.

radiologist
A doctor who's an expert in reading imaging tests—tests that make pictures of the inside of the body.

rectum
The last part of the large intestine that holds stool until it's expelled from the body.

recurrence
The return of cancer after treatment. Also called a relapse.

recurrence treatment
Treatment that is given after prior treatments failed to kill all the cancer or keep it away.

regimen
A treatment plan that specifies the drug(s), dose, schedule, and length of treatment.

relapse
The return of cancer after treatment. Also called a recurrence.

reproductive organs
Organs that help make babies.

reproductive system
The group of organs that work together to make babies. In women, this includes the ovaries, fallopian tubes, uterus, cervix, and vagina.

serous
The most common cell subtype of ovarian cancer.

side effect
An unhealthy or unpleasant condition caused by treatment.

sigmoid colon
The last part of the colon—organ that changes unused food from a liquid to a solid form—that connects to the rectum, which holds stool until it leaves the body.

small intestine
The digestive organ that absorbs nutrients from eaten food.

spleen
An organ to the left of the stomach that helps protect the body from disease.

stromal cell
Cells that form the connective and supporting tissues that hold the ovary together.

sugar radiotracer
A form of sugar that is put into your body and lets off a small amount of energy that is absorbed by active cells.

supportive care
Treatment given to relieve the symptoms of a disease. Also called palliative care.

surgeon
A doctor who is an expert in operations to remove or repair a part of the body.

surgery
An operation to remove or repair a part of the body.

surgical staging
The process of finding out how far cancer has spread by performing tests and procedures during surgery to remove the cancer.

surgical treatment
Treatment with surgery—an operation to remove or repair a part of the body.

symptom
A new or changed health problem a person experiences that may indicate a certain disease or health condition.

targeted therapy
Treatment with drugs that target a specific or unique feature of cancer cells.

Dictionary

taxane
A type of cancer drug that blocks certain cell parts to stop a cell from dividing into two cells.

treatment plan
A written course of action through cancer treatment and beyond.

treatment response
An outcome or improvement related to treatment.

tumor
An abnormal mass formed by the overgrowth of cells.

tumor marker
A substance found in body tissue or fluid that may be a sign of cancer.

U.S. Food and Drug Administration
A federal government agency that regulates drugs and food in the United States.

ultrasound
A test that uses sound waves to take pictures of the inside of the body.

unilateral salpingo-oophorectomy (USO)
Surgery that removes one ovary and the attached fallopian tube.

uterus
The female organ where babies grow during pregnancy. Also called womb.

vagina
The hollow, muscular tube in women through which babies are born.

vein
A blood vessel that carries blood back to the heart from all parts of the body.

washings
Sample of liquid that is tested for cancer cells after it is used to "wash" the inside of the belly (peritoneal cavity).

white blood cell
A type of blood cell that helps fight infections in the body.

Acronyms

NCCN®
National Comprehensive Cancer Network®

AJCC
American Joint Committee on Cancer

AFP
alpha-fetoprotein

BEP
bleomycin, etoposide, and cisplatin

BSO
bilateral salpingo-oophorectomy

CA-125
cancer antigen 125

CAM
complementary and alternative medicine

CBC
complete blood count

CEA
carcinoembryonic antigen

cm
centimeter

CT
computed tomography

DNA
deoxyribonucleic acid

FDA
U.S. Food and Drug Administration

FIGO
International Federation of Gynecology and Obstetrics

FNA
fine-needle aspiration

GI
gastrointestinal

HNPCC
heredity non-polyposis colorectal cancer syndrome

IP
intraperitoneal

IV
intravenous

LCOH
less common ovarian histopathologies

LHRH
luteinizing hormone-releasing hormone

LMP
low malignant potential

mm
millimeter

MMMT
malignant mixed Müllerian tumor

MRI
magnetic resonance imaging

PARP
poly ADP-ribose polymerase

PET
positron emission tomography

PET/CT
positron emission tomography/computed tomography

TAH
total abdominal hysterectomy

TKI
tyrosine kinase inhibitor

USO
unilateral salpingo-oophorectomy

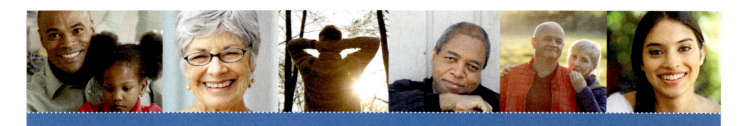

State Fundraising Notices

FLORIDA: A COPY OF THE OFFICIAL REGISTRATION AND FINANCIAL INFORMATION OF NCCN FOUNDATION MAY BE OBTAINED FROM THE DIVISION OF CONSUMER SERVICES BY CALLING TOLL-FREE WITHIN THE STATE 1-800-HELP-FLA. REGISTRATION DOES NOT IMPLY ENDORSEMENT, APPROVAL, OR RECOMMENDATION BY THE STATE. FLORIDA REGISTRATION #CH33263. **GEORGIA:** The following information will be sent upon request: (A) A full and fair description of the programs and activities of NCCN Foundation; and (B) A financial statement or summary which shall be consistent with the financial statement required to be filed with the Secretary of State pursuant to Code Section 43-17-5. **KANSAS:** The annual financial report for NCCN Foundation, 275 Commerce Drive, Suite 300, Fort Washington, PA 19034, 215-690-0300, State Registration # 445-497-1, is filed with the Secretary of State. **MARYLAND:** A copy of the NCCN Foundation financial report is available by calling NCCN Foundation at 215-690-0300 or writing to 275 Commerce Drive, Suite 300, Fort Washington, PA 19034. For the cost of copying and postage, documents and information filed under the Maryland charitable organizations law can be obtained from the Secretary of State, Charitable Division, State House, Annapolis, MD 21401, 1-410-974-5534. **MICHIGAN:** Registration Number MICS 45298. **MISSISSIPPI:** The official registration and financial information of NCCN Foundation may be obtained from the Mississippi Secretary of State's office by calling 888-236-6167. Registration by the Secretary of State does not imply endorsement by the Secretary of State. **NEW JERSEY:** INFORMATION FILED WITH THE ATTORNEY GENERAL CONCERNING THIS CHARITABLE SOLICITATION AND THE PERCENTAGE OF CONTRIBUTIONS RECEIVED BY THE CHARITY DURING THE LAST REPORTING PERIOD THAT WERE DEDICATED TO THE CHARITABLE PURPOSE MAY BE OBTAINED FROM THE ATTORNEY GENERAL OF THE STATE OF NEW JERSEY BY CALLING (973) 504-6215 AND IS AVAILABLE ON THE INTERNET AT www.njconsumeraffairs.gov/ocp.htm#charity. REGISTRATION WITH THE ATTORNEY GENERAL DOES NOT IMPLY ENDORSEMENT. **NEW YORK:** A copy of the latest annual report may be obtained from NCCN Foundation, 275 Commerce Drive, Suite 300, Fort Washington, PA 19034, or the Charities Bureau, Department of Law. 120 Broadway, New York, NY 10271. **NORTH CAROLINA: FINANCIAL INFORMATION ABOUT THIS ORGANIZATION AND A COPY OF ITS LICENSE ARE AVAILABLE FROM THE STATE SOLICITATION LICENSING BRANCH AT 888-830-4989 (within North Carolina) or (919) 807-2214 (outside of North Carolina). THE LICENSE IS NOT AN ENDORSEMENT BY THE STATE. PENNSYLVANIA:** The official registration and financial information of NCCN Foundation may be obtained from the Pennsylvania Department of State by calling toll-free within Pennsylvania, 800-732-0999. Registration does not imply endorsement. **VIRGINIA:** A financial statement for the most recent fiscal year is available upon request from the State Division of Consumer Affairs, P.O. Box 1163, Richmond, VA 23218; 1-804-786-1343. **WASHINGTON:** Our charity is registered with the Secretary of State and information relating to our financial affairs is available from the Secretary of State, toll free for Washington residents 800-332-4483. **WEST VIRGINIA:** West Virginia residents may obtain a summary of the registration and financial documents from the Secretary of State, State Capitol, Charleston, WV 25305. Registration does not imply endorsement.

Consult with the IRS or your tax professional regarding tax deductibility. REGISTRATION OR LICENSING WITH A STATE AGENCY DOES NOT CONSTITUTE OR IMPLY ENDORSEMENT, APPROVAL, OR RECOMMENDATION BY THAT STATE. We care about your privacy and how we communicate with you, and how we use and share your information. For a copy of NCCN Foundation's Privacy Policy, please call 215.690.0300 or visit our website at www.nccn.org.

NCCN Panel Members for Ovarian Cancer

Robert J. Morgan, Jr., MD/Chair
City of Hope Comprehensive Cancer Center

Deborah K. Armstrong, MD/Interim Vice Chair
The Sidney Kimmel Comprehensive Cancer Center at Johns Hopkins

Steven C. Plaxe, MD/Interim Vice Chair
UC San Diego Moores Cancer Center

Ronald D. Alvarez, MD
Vanderbilt-Ingram Cancer Center

Jamie N. Bakkum-Gamez, MD
Mayo Clinic Cancer Center

Lisa Barroilhet, MD
University of Wisconsin Carbone Cancer Center

Kian Behbakht, MD
University of Colorado Cancer Center

Lee-may Chen, MD
UCSF Helen Diller Family Comprehensive Cancer Center

Marta Ann Crispens, MD
Vanderbilt-Ingram Cancer Center

Maria DeRosa, RN

Oliver Dorigo, MD, PhD
Stanford Cancer Institute

David M. Gershenson, MD
The University of Texas MD Anderson Cancer Center

Heidi J. Gray, MD
University of Washington Medical Center/ Seattle Cancer Care Alliance

Ardeshir Hakam, MD
Moffitt Cancer Center

Laura J. Havrilesky, MD
Duke Cancer Institute

Carolyn Johnston, MD
University of Michigan Comprehensive Cancer Center

Monica B. Jones, MD
Duke Cancer Institute

Charles A. Leath III, MD
University of Alabama at Birmingham Comprehensive Cancer Center

Shashikant Lele, MD
Roswell Park Cancer Institute

Lainie Martin, MD
Fox Chase Cancer Center

Ursula A. Matulonis, MD
Dana-Farber/Brigham and Women's Cancer Center

David M. O'Malley, MD
The Ohio State University Comprehensive Cancer Center - James Cancer Hospital and Solove Research Institute

Richard T. Penson, MD, MRCP
Massachusetts General Hospital Cancer Center

Sanja Percac-Lima, MD
Massachusetts General Hospital Cancer Center

Mario Pineda, MD, PhD
Robert H. Lurie Comprehensive Cancer Center of Northwestern University

Matthew A. Powell, MD
Siteman Cancer Center at Barnes-Jewish Hospital and Washington University School of Medicine

Elena Ratner, MD
Yale Cancer Center/Smilow Cancer Hospital

Steven W. Remmenga, MD
Fred & Pamela Buffett Cancer Center

Peter G. Rose, MD
Case Comprehensive Cancer Center/ University Hospitals Seidman Cancer Center and Cleveland Clinic Taussig Cancer Institute

Paul Sabbatini, MD
Memorial Sloan Kettering Cancer Center

Joseph T. Santoso, MD
St. Jude Children's Research Hospital/ The University of Tennessee Health Science Center

Theresa L. Werner, MD
Huntsman Cancer Institute at the University of Utah

NCCN Staff

Jennifer Burns
Guidelines Coordinator

Miranda Hughes, PhD
Oncology Scientist/Senior Medical Writer

For disclosures, visit www.nccn.org/about/disclosure.aspx.

NCCN Member Institutions

Fred & Pamela Buffett Cancer Center
Omaha, Nebraska
800.999.5465
nebraskamed.com/cancer

**Case Comprehensive Cancer Center/
University Hospitals Seidman
Cancer Center and Cleveland Clinic
Taussig Cancer Institute**
Cleveland, Ohio
800.641.2422 • UH Seidman Cancer Center
uhhospitals.org/seidman
866.223.8100 • CC Taussig Cancer Institute
my.clevelandclinic.org/services/cancer
216.844.8797 • Case CCC
case.edu/cancer

**City of Hope Comprehensive
Cancer Center**
Los Angeles, California
800.826.4673
cityofhope.org

**Dana-Farber/Brigham and
Women's Cancer Center
Massachusetts General Hospital
Cancer Center**
Boston, Massachusetts
877.332.4294
dfbwcc.org
massgeneral.org/cancer

Duke Cancer Institute
Durham, North Carolina
888.275.3853
dukecancerinstitute.org

Fox Chase Cancer Center
Philadelphia, Pennsylvania
888.369.2427
foxchase.org

**Huntsman Cancer Institute
at the University of Utah**
Salt Lake City, Utah
877.585.0303
huntsmancancer.org

**Fred Hutchinson Cancer
Research Center/
Seattle Cancer Care Alliance**
Seattle, Washington
206.288.7222 • seattlecca.org
206.667.5000 • fredhutch.org

**The Sidney Kimmel Comprehensive
Cancer Center at Johns Hopkins**
Baltimore, Maryland
410.955.8964
hopkinskimmelcancercenter.org

**Robert H. Lurie Comprehensive Cancer
Center of Northwestern University**
Chicago, Illinois
866.587.4322
cancer.northwestern.edu

Mayo Clinic Cancer Center
Phoenix/Scottsdale, Arizona
Jacksonville, Florida
Rochester, Minnesota
800.446.2279 • Arizona
904.953.0853 • Florida
507.538.3270 • Minnesota
mayoclinic.org/departments-centers/mayo-clinic-cancer-center

**Memorial Sloan Kettering
Cancer Center**
New York, New York
800.525.2225
mskcc.org

Moffitt Cancer Center
Tampa, Florida
800.456.3434
moffitt.org

**The Ohio State University
Comprehensive Cancer Center -
James Cancer Hospital and
Solove Research Institute**
Columbus, Ohio
800.293.5066
cancer.osu.edu

Roswell Park Cancer Institute
Buffalo, New York
877.275.7724
roswellpark.org

**Siteman Cancer Center at Barnes-
Jewish Hospital and Washington
University School of Medicine**
St. Louis, Missouri
800.600.3606
siteman.wustl.edu

**St. Jude Children's Research Hospital
The University of Tennessee
Health Science Center**
Memphis, Tennessee
888.226.4343 • stjude.org
901.683.0055 • westclinic.com

Stanford Cancer Institute
Stanford, California
877.668.7535
cancer.stanford.edu

**University of Alabama at Birmingham
Comprehensive Cancer Center**
Birmingham, Alabama
800.822.0933
www3.ccc.uab.edu

UC San Diego Moores Cancer Center
La Jolla, California
858.657.7000
cancer.ucsd.edu

**UCSF Helen Diller Family
Comprehensive Cancer Center**
San Francisco, California
800.689.8273
cancer.ucsf.edu

University of Colorado Cancer Center
Aurora, Colorado
720.848.0300
coloradocancercenter.org

**University of Michigan
Comprehensive Cancer Center**
Ann Arbor, Michigan
800.865.1125
mcancer.org

**The University of Texas
MD Anderson Cancer Center**
Houston, Texas
800.392.1611
mdanderson.org

Vanderbilt-Ingram Cancer Center
Nashville, Tennessee
800.811.8480
vicc.org

**University of Wisconsin
Carbone Cancer Center**
Madison, Wisconsin
608.265.1700
uwhealth.org/cancer

**Yale Cancer Center/
Smilow Cancer Hospital**
New Haven, Connecticut
855.4.SMILOW
yalecancercenter.org

Index

adjuvant treatment 37, 50, 54, 65–72, 74, 78

biopsy 14, 21, 23–24, 46–48, 51–53, 70

blood test 14, 20–21, 55–56, 58, 67–68, 72, 75, 77, 80

borderline epithelial tumors (LMP [low malignant potential] 10, 12, 70–73

CA-125 14, 20, 50, 55–56, 58–60, 72–73, 75, 80

carcinosarcoma (MMMT [malignant mixed Müllerian tumor] 10, 64–65

cancer grade 30, 32, 47–48, 50

cancer stage 22–23, 23–29, 32, 45–54, 65

chemotherapy 30, 32, 35, 37–42, 47–50, 52–56, 59–60, 62, 65–70, 72–74, 77–79

clear cell carcinoma of the ovary 66

clinical trial 30, 41–42, 56–57, 59–60, 65, 75, 85

completion surgery 47–48, 52, 54, 58, 66, 68, 70–72, 76–77

debulking surgery 35–36, 51, 73, 75

fertility-sparing surgery 35, 46, 58, 66–72, 74, 76–77

follow-up test 49–50, 56, 58, 60, 65, 70, 72–73, 80

genetic counseling 14–15, 21, 60

hormone therapy 40–42, 62, 66, 69

imaging test 14, 16–19, 21, 50, 55–56, 58–60, 73, 75, 77, 80

implant 10, 26, 70–73

intraperitoneal (IP) chemotherapy 38–39, 55

intravenous (IV) chemotherapy 38–39, 50, 55

low-grade (grade 1) serous/endometrioid epithelial carcinoma 68–69

malignant germ cell tumor 10, 76–80

malignant sex cord-stromal tumor 68, 74–75, 80

mucinous carcinoma of the ovary 67–68

primary chemotherapy 37, 50, 54, 56

primary treatment 35, 37, 42, 45–48, 50–54, 68, 70, 72–73, 76

recurrence 56–57, 59–62, 65, 73, 75, 80

recurrence treatment 56–57, 59–62, 65, 75

relapse 58–60, 62, 73, 75

reproductive 8, 23, 30, 35

side effect 20, 31, 37, 39–42, 50, 55, 57–58, 60

supportive care 56–57, 59–60

surgery 14, 21, 23–24, 26, 30, 32, 35–37, 39, 42, 45–55, 58–79

surgical staging 23–24, 32, 36, 45–48, 50–52, 60, 65–68, 70–72, 76–77

symptom 12, 14–15, 31–32, 37, 41, 57, 60, 65, 73, 75

targeted therapy 39–40, 42, 62

treatment response 55–56, 62

Made in the USA
Lexington, KY
22 February 2018